Vegan Mostly Alkaline

Compiled by
Bro. D. Clement El

Edited by
Sis. T. Najee-Ullah El

© 2024
Califa Media™

Vegan Mostly Alkaline

by

Bro. D. Clement El

©2024 Califa Media

ISBN 13: 978-1-952828-26-3

All Rights Reserved. Without Prejudice. No Part Of This Book May Be Reproduced Or Transmitted In Any Form By Any Means, Electronic, Photocopying, Mechanical, Recording, Information Storage Or Retrieval System Unless For The Liberation Of Minds And Gaining Knowledge Of Self.

COPYRIGHT DISCLAIMER: *Under Sec.107 OF THE COPYRIGHT ACT OF 1976, allowance is made for "fair use" for purposes such as criticism, comment, news reporting, teaching, scholarship, and research. Fair use is permitted by copyright statute that might otherwise be infringing. Non-profit, educational, or personal use tips the balance in favor of fair use.*

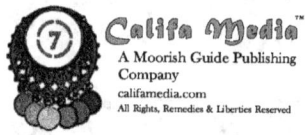

Califa Media
A Moorish Guide Publishing Company
califamedia.com
All Rights, Remedies & Liberties Reserved

Contents

Chapter 1: Shopping List — 1
- Fruits 2
- Vegetables 3
- Teas, Sweeteners, & Spices — 4
- Nuts, Seeds, & Oils 5
- pH Chart 6
- Kitchen Tools 8

Chapter 2: Soups & Sauces — 9
- Chili 11
- Veggie Soup (Not Chicken) — 12
- Brown Sauce (Manchurian) — 13
- Red Sauce 14
- Creamy Alfredo Sauce 16
- Pesto 17
- Tzatziki 18
- Garlic Tahini 19
- Guacamole 20
- Salsa (Pico de Gallo) 21
- Jerk Sauce (Marinade) 22

Chapter 3: Sides & Starters — 23
- Pasta / Potato Salad Dressing 24
- Slaw 25
- Hummus 26
- Simple House Dressing — 27
- Seaweed Salad (Wakame) — 28
- Simple Veggie Sautés 29

Chapter 4: Indigenous Rices & Grains — 30
- Garlic Turmeric Rice 31
- Indigenous American Rice (Arroz con Gandules) 32
- Fried Rice (Manchurian) — 33
- Burro Fries / Fried Plantain — 34

Chapter 5: Entrees — 37
- Pancakes / Waffles 38
- Falafel 40
- BBQ Jackfruit 42
- Jackfruit Tuna/Chicken — 44
- Jackfruit Veggie Tacos / Burritos 46
- Jerk Veggies 48
- Asiatic Mixed Veggies 50
- Noodles in Brown Sauce — 52
- Pastas (Red Sauce, Creamy Alfredo, Pesto) 54
- Crab Cake (Lions Mane Mushroom) 56
- Pizza / Flatbread 58
- Chopped Cheese 60
- Wraps / Sandwiches 62

Chapter 6: Sips & Sweets — 64
- Tamarindo 65
- Hibiscus (Sorrel) 66
- Limeade 67
- Seamoss Smoothies 68
- Banana Bread / Muffins / Donuts 70
- Raw Strawberry Cheesecake Donuts 72
- Peanut Butter Dates 74
- Other Titles from Califa Media 75

Notes

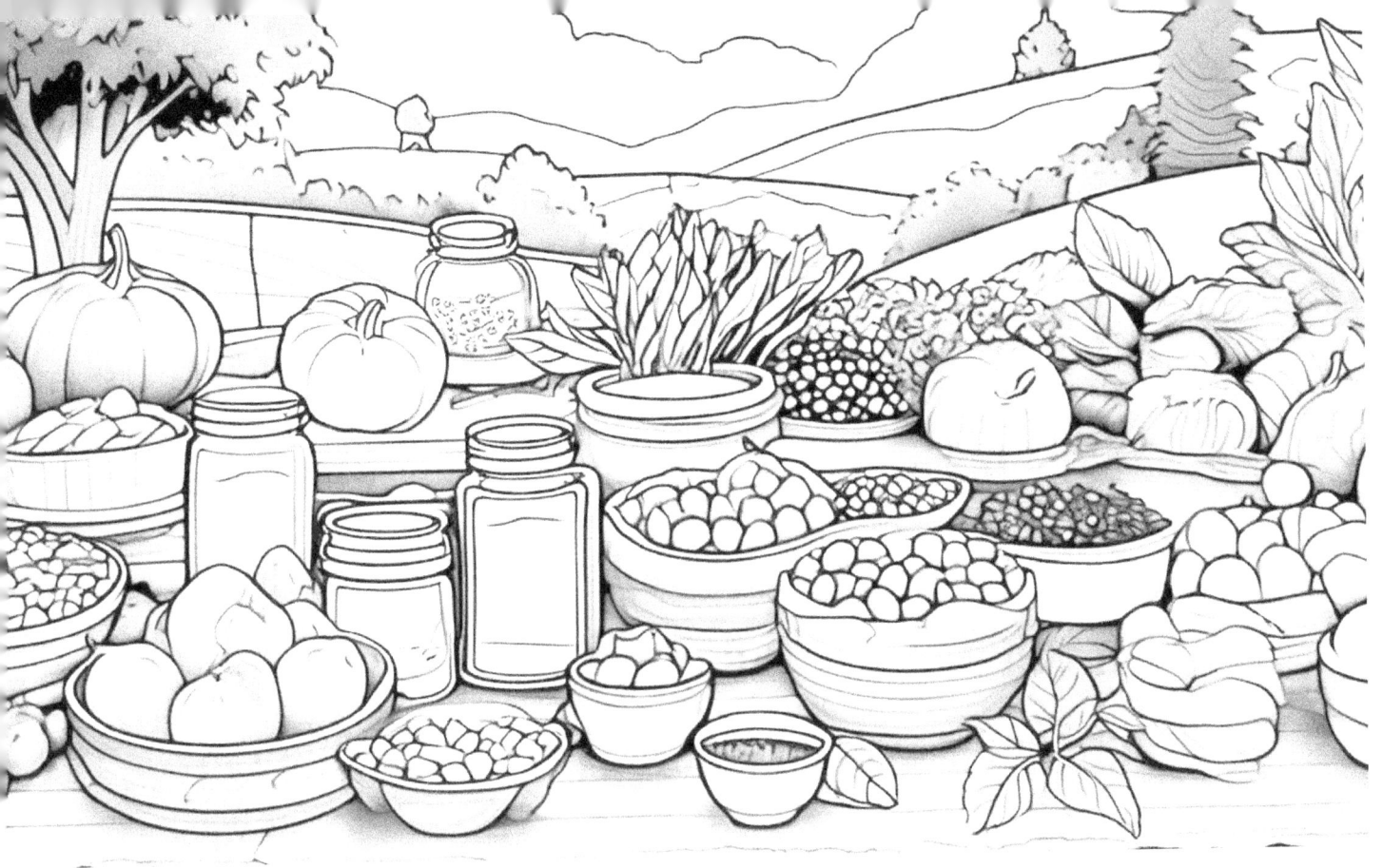

1. SHOPPING LIST

Before we get started, as with any project, first we must gather our supplies. This chapter provides a comprehensive shopping list for stocking a vegan kitchen and pantry. It covers all the essential fruits, vegetables, teas, seasonings, nuts, seeds, and oils needed for preparing delicious plant-based meals. Understanding the pH levels of various foods is crucial for maintaining an alkaline balance in the body. The chapter includes an extensive reference table detailing the approximate pH values of common ingredients like fruits, vegetables, vinegars, and more. Having this knowledge allows you to make informed choices when meal planning. In addition to the shopping lists, there are recommendations for must-have kitchen tools and equipment. From high-powered blenders for silky smoothies to durable stainless steel cookware, these tools will enable you to fully embrace the vegan lifestyle. With this chapter as a guide, you'll be well-equipped to shop for and prepare vibrant, healthy vegan dishes.

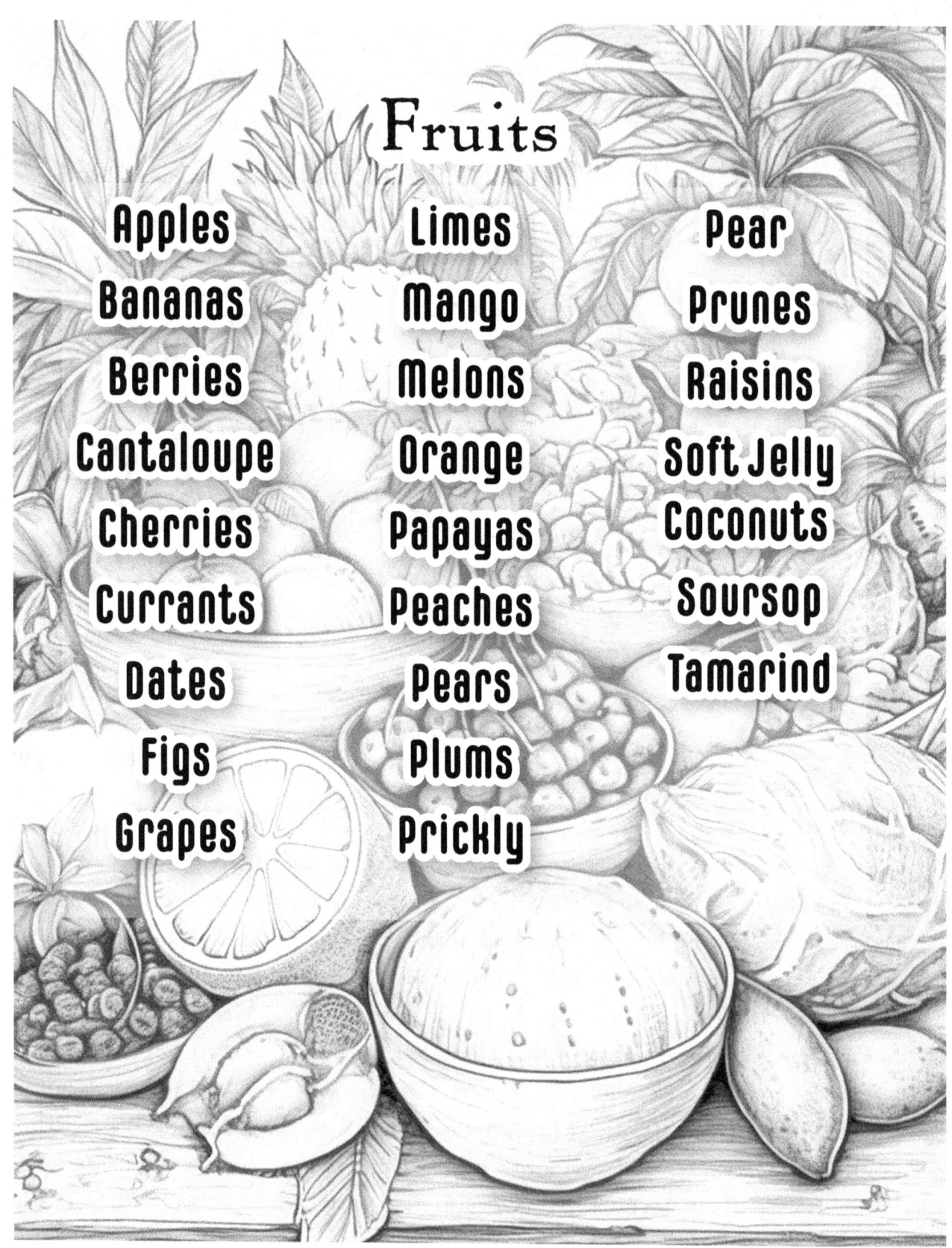

Fruits

- Apples
- Bananas
- Berries
- Cantaloupe
- Cherries
- Currants
- Dates
- Figs
- Grapes
- Limes
- Mango
- Melons
- Orange
- Papayas
- Peaches
- Pears
- Plums
- Prickly
- Pear
- Prunes
- Raisins
- Soft Jelly Coconuts
- Soursop
- Tamarind

Ch 2: Soups + Sauces : Fruits

Vegetables

- Amaranth
- Arame
- Avocado
- Bell Pepper
- Chayote
- Cherry and Plum Tomato
- Cucumber
- Dandelion Greens
- Dulse
- Garbanzo Beans
- Hijiki
- Izote flower and leaf
- Kale
- Lettuce (except Iceberg)
- Mushrooms (except Shiitake)
- Nopales
- Nori
- Okra
- Olives
- Onions
- Purslane
- Verdolaga
- Squash
- Tomatillo
- Turnip Greens
- Wakame
- Watercress
- Wild Arugula
- Zucchini

Teas, Sweetners and Spices

- Burdock
- Chamomile
- Elderberry
- Fennel
- Ginger
- Red Raspberry
- Tila
- Date Sugar (from dried dates)
- 100% Pure Agave Syrup (from cactus)

- Achiote
- Basil
- Bay Leaf
- Cayenne
- Cloves
- Dill
- Habanero
- Onion Powder
- Oregano

- Powdered Granulated Seaweed
- Pure Sea Salt
- Sage
- Savory
- Sweet Basil
- Tarragon
- Thyme

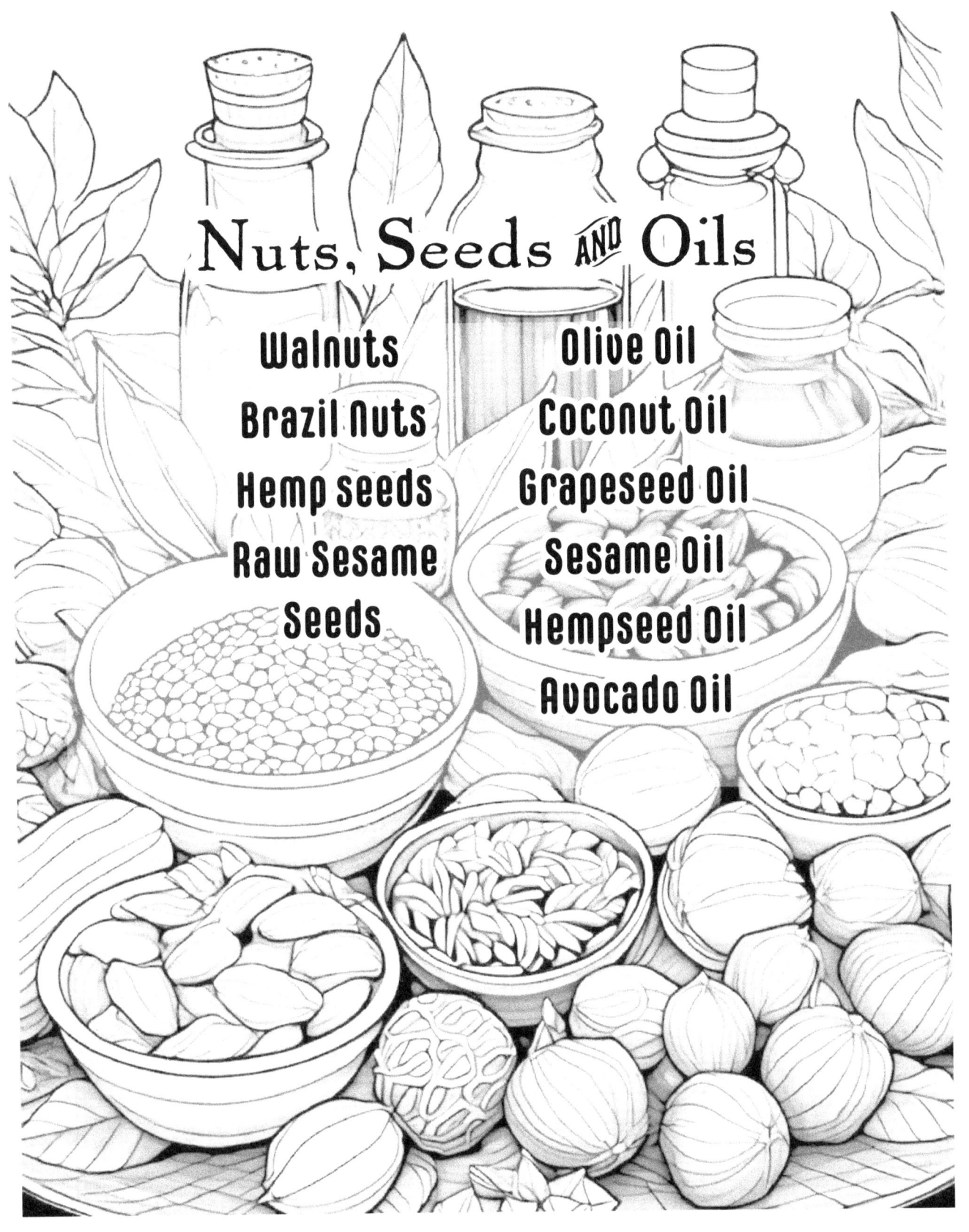

pH Values

Maintaining a balanced pH level in your body is crucial for optimal health. Many plant-based foods are naturally alkaline-forming, helping to neutralize acidity and reduce inflammation. It's important to include a variety of fruits and veggies to ensure you're getting a well-rounded intake of nutrients. Alkaline water, with a higher pH level, can provide additional benefits by neutralizing acid in the body and enhancing hydration.

Item	Approx. pH	Item	Approx. pH
Apple, baked with sugar	3.20 - 3.55	Broccoli	6.30-6.85
Apple, eating	3.30-4.00	Brussels sprout	6.00-6.30
Apple - Delicious	3.9	Cabbage	5.20-6.8
Apple - Golden Delicious	3.6	Cabbage, green	5.50-6.75
Apple - Jonathan	3.33	Cactus	4.70
Apple - McIntosh	3.34	Cantaloupe	6.13-6.58
Apple Juice	3.35-4.00	Carrots	5.88-6.40
Apple Sauce	3.10-3.60	Cauliflower	5.6
Apple - Winesap	3.47	Celery	5.70-6.00
Apricots	3.30-4.80	Cherries, California	4.01-4.54
Apricot nectar	3.78	Cherries, red, water pack	3.25-3.82
Apricots, pureed	3.42-3.83	Cherries, Royal Ann	3.80-3.83
Artichokes	5.50-6.00	Corn	5.90-7.50
Artichokes, canned, acidified	4.30-4.60	Cucumbers	5.12-5.78
Artichokes, Jerusalem, cooked	5.93-6.00	Cucumbers, dill pickles	3.20-3.70
Asparagus	6.00-6.70	Cucumbers, pickled	4.20-4.60
Avocados	6.27-6.58	Eggplant	4.5-5.3
Baby corn	5.20	Figs, Calamyrna	5.05-5.98
Bamboo Shoots	5.10-6.20	Four bean salad	5.60
Bananas	4.50-5.20	Fruit cocktaii	3.60-4.00
Beans	5.60-6.50	Grapes, Concord	2.80-3.00
Beans, black	5.78-6.02	Grapes, Niagara	2.80-3.27
Beans, kidney	5.40-6.00	Grapes, seedless	2.90-3.82
Beans, lima	6.50	Grapefruit	3.00-3.75
Beans, soy	6.00-6.60	Horseradish, ground	5.35
Beans, string	5.60	Jam,.fruit	3.50-4.50
Beans, wax	5.30-5.70	Jellies, fruit	3.00-3.50
Beans, pork & tomato sauce	5.10-5.80	Ketchup	3.89-3.92
Beets	5.30-6.60	Leeks	5.50-6.17
Beets, canned, acidified	4.30-4.60	Lemon juice	2.00-2.60
Blackberries, Washington	3.85-4.50	Lime juiice	2.00-2.35
Blueberriies, Maine	3.12-3.33	Lime	2.00-2.80
Blueberries, frozen	3.11-3.22	Loganberries	2.70-3.50

Common Ingredients

Butter	6.1 - 6.4	Cornstarch	4.0 - 7.0	Corn Syrup	5.0	Flour	6.0 - 6.3
Honey	3.9	Molasses	5.0 - 5.5	Sugar	5.0-6.0	Vinegar	2.0 -3.4

Item	Approx. pH	Item	Approx. pH
Mangoes, ripe	5..80-6.00	Pimiento	4.40-4.90
Mangoes, green	3..40-4.80	Pineapple	3.20-4.00
Maple syrup	5.15	Plums, Blue	2.80-3.40
Melon, Honey dew	6.00-6.67	Plums, Red	3.60-4.30
Mint jelly	3.01	Pomegranate	2.93-3.20
Mushrooms	6.00-6.70	Potatoes	5.40-5.90
Nectarines	3.92-4.18	Prunes	3.63-3.92
Okra, cooked	5.50-6.60	Pumpkin	4.990-5.50
Olives, black	6.00-7.00	Radishes, red	5.85-6.05
Olives, green fermented	3.60-4.60	Radishes, white	5.52-5.69
Olives, ripe	6.00-7.50	Raspberries	3.22-3.95
Onions, pickled	3.70-4.60	Rhubarb	3.10-3.40
Onions, red	5.30-5.880	Sauerkraut	3.30-3.60
Onions, white	5.37-5.85	Spinach	5.50-6.80
Onions, yellow	5.32-5.60	Squash, acorn, cooked	5.18-6.49
Oranges, Florida	3.69-4.34	Squash, white, cooked	5.52-5.80
Orange juice, California	3.30-4.19	Squash, yellow, cooked	5.79-6.00
Orange juice, Florida	3.30-4.15	Strawberries	3.00-3.90
Palm, heart of	6.70	Sweet potatoes	5.30-5.60
Papaya	5.20-6.00	Tofu (soybean curd)	7.20
Parsnip	5.30-5.70	Tomatillo	3.83
Peaches	3.30-4.05	Tomatoes	4.30-4.90
Pears, Bartlett	3.50-4.60	Tomatoes, juice	4.10-4.60
Peas, canned	5.70-6.00	Tomatoes, paste	3.50-4.70
Peas, Garbanzo	6.48-6.80	Tomatoes, vine ripened	4.42-4.65
Peppers	4.65-5.45	Vinegar	2.40-3.40
Peppers, green	5.20-5.93	Vinegar, cider	3.10
Persimmons	4.42-4.70	Watermelon	5.18-5.60
Pickles, fresh pack	5..10-5.40	Zucchini, cooked	5.69-6.10

References:

Anon. 1962. pH values of food products. Food Eng. 34(3): 98-99.
Bridges, M.A., and Mattice, M.R. 1939. Over two thousand estimations of the pH of representative foods, American J. Digestive Diseases, 9:440-449.
Warren L. Landry, et al. 1995. Examination of canned foods. FDA BAM, AOAC International.
Grahn M.A. 1984. Acidified and low acid foods from Southeast Asia. FDA-LIB

Kitchen Tools

- High power blender (for soups and sauces)
- Food processor
- Cast iron pots (Dutch Oven)
- Pans
- Wok
- Grill flat top
- Glass (vintage Pyrex) pots and pans.
- Stainless steel pots and pans (perfect for cooking on induction style burners)
- Stainless steel cooking utensils including knives, measuring cups & spoons, whisks, grill spatulas, scraper, funnels, strainers
- Silicone bowl scrapers and spatula

GALLON	QUART	PINT	CUP	OUNCE	TBLSP	TSP	mL	DROP
1	4	8	16	128	256	768	3,840	79,800
	1	2	4	32	64	192	960	19,200
		1	2	16	32	96	480	9,600
			1	8	16	48	240	4,800
				1	2	6	30	600
					1	3	15	300
						1	5	100
							1	20

Ch 2: Soups + Sauces : pH Values

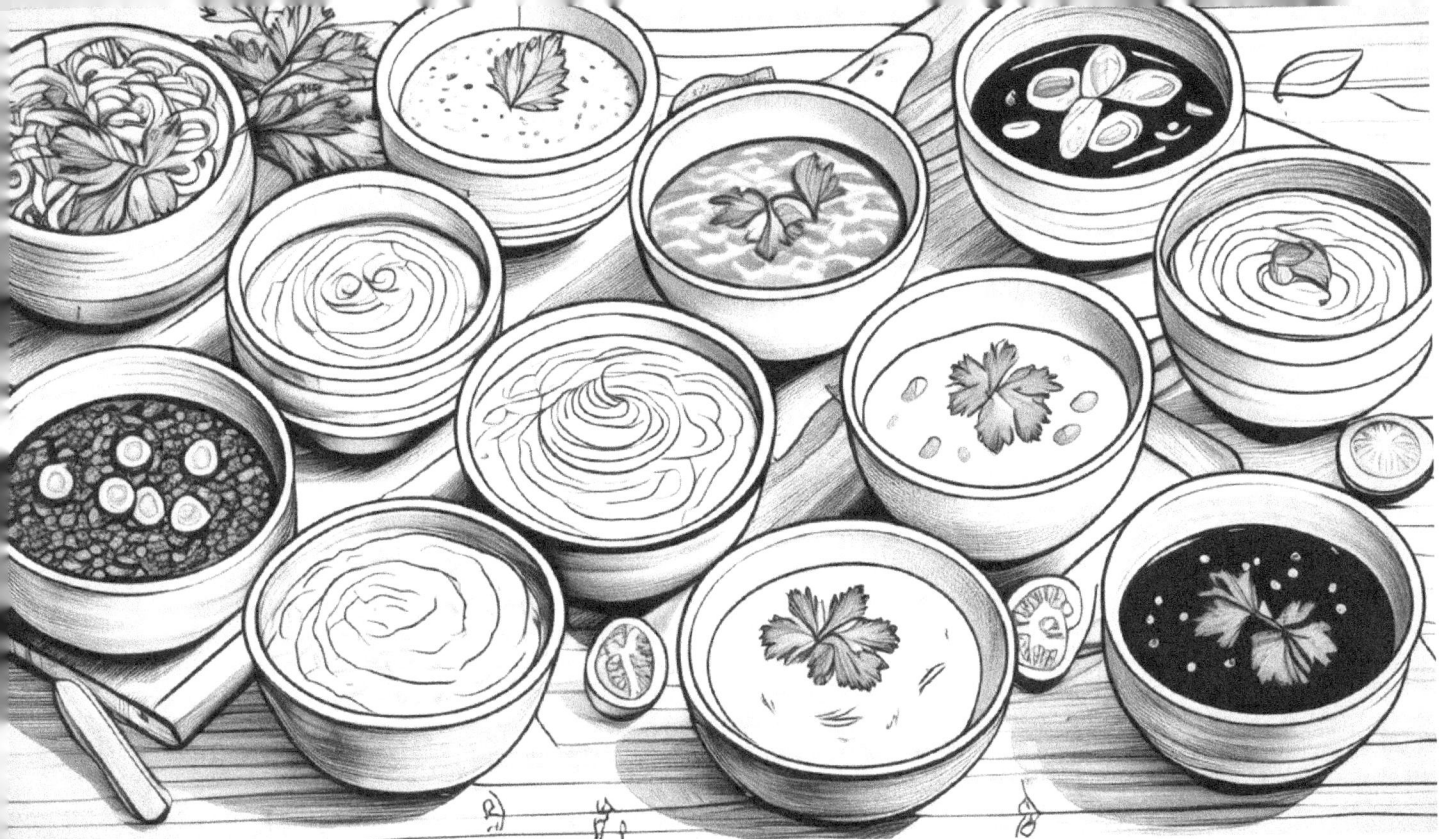

2.
SOUPS
{AND}
SAUCES

I remember receiving advice that the key to success in the kitchen/restaurant business is developing soups and sauces. In the years since then, I have come to realize the truth in that statement. One cannot resist a good bowl of soup. Soups are inexpensive when prepared based on the portions of serving—they can be served as both an appetizer and an entree, which makes them versatile to serve several people for quite a while. The longer they stay in the refrigerator, the better they become. Sauces, in my experience, are the base of almost every great dish I have ever tasted.

So let's start our recipe base with the very base of every recipe: Soups + Sauces.

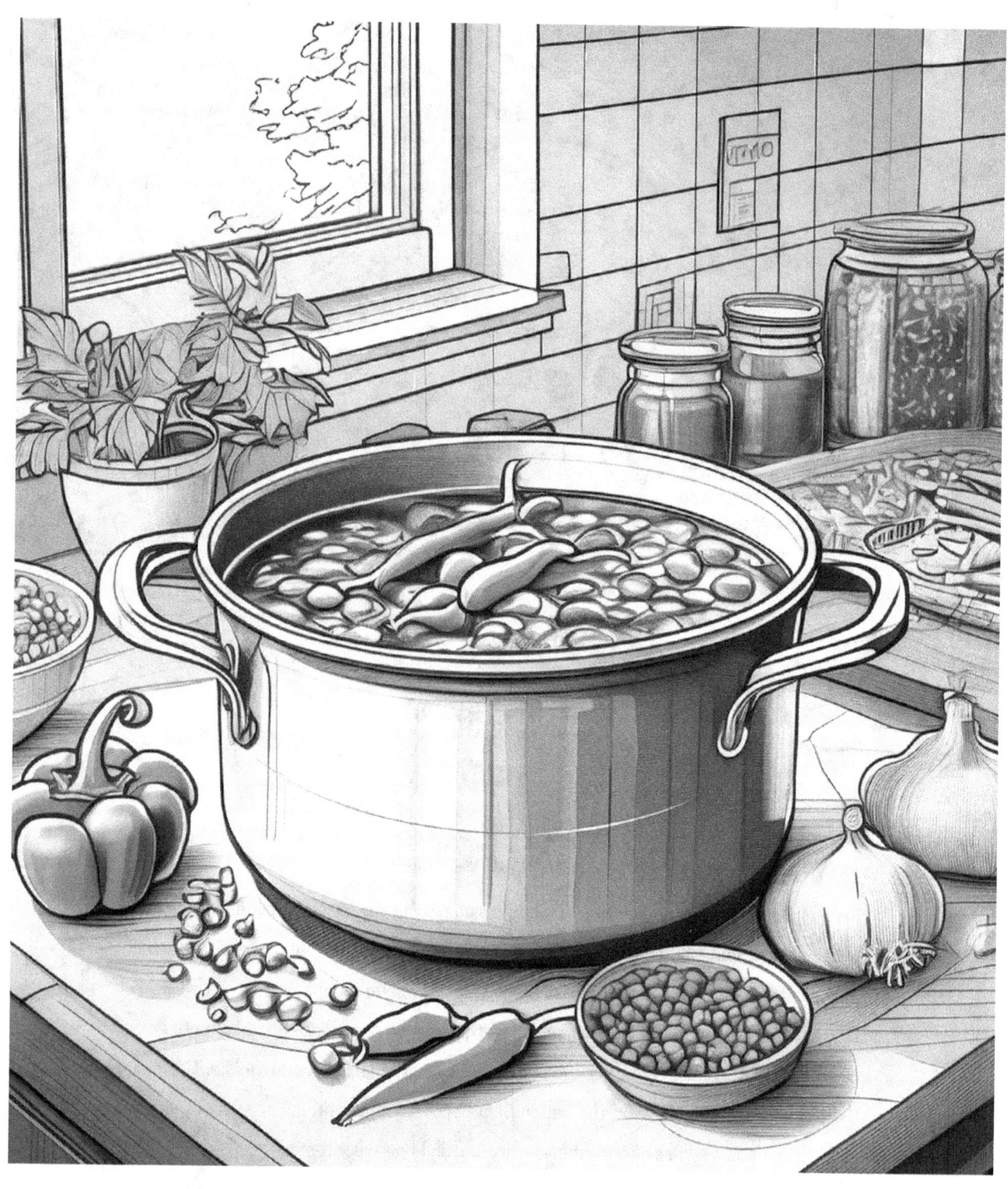

Ch 2: Soups + Sauces : Chili

Chili

From its roots in indigenous America to its rise as a popular classic, Chili shows an amazing fusion of culinary traditions in world cuisines. This vegan chili speaks to that legacy and provides plant-based ingredients that echo the respect for nature in their innovation. Using a multitude of flavors, this recipe modernizes an ancient and venerable tradition while at the same time keeping health and sustainability in mind. It also offers an opening to a broad audience to peer deeper into American cuisine and, through food, it unites cultures. This style of chili really brings the world of communities together by serving a taste of common heritage.

Ingredients

- 2 large onion, diced
- 2 large red bell pepper, diced
- 2 large green bell pepper diced 5 cloves minced garlic
- 1 splash vegetable broth (for sautéing)
- 8 Oz your choice of meat substitutes (OR) 8 Oz can tomato sauce
- 15 oz can fire-roasted diced tomatoes
- 4 Cups vegetable broth
- ¼ Cup McCormick's chili powder 2 Tsp ground cumin
- 1 Tsp smoked paprika 1 Tsp oregano
- 15 Oz can garbanzo beans (drained & rinsed)) 15 Oz can kidney beans (not drained)
- ½ Tsp black pepper
- ½ Tsp garlic powder
- 2 Tbsp pickled jalapeños (optional)

Nutrition Facts

Serving size: 1 cup
Servings: 8

Amount per serving

Calories 449

	% Daily Value*
Total Fat 16.3g	21%
Saturated Fat 1.9g	9%
Cholesterol 0mg	0%
Sodium 1494mg	65%
Total Carbohydrate 58.7g	21%
Dietary Fiber 21.5g	77%
Total Sugars 11.6g	
Protein 28.4g	
Vitamin D 0mcg	0%
Calcium 394mg	30%
Iron 27mg	151%
Potassium 2144mg	46%

*The % Daily Value (DV) tells you how much a nutrient in a food serving contributes to a daily diet. 2,000 calorie a day is used for general nutrition advice.

Recipe analyzed by **well**

Instructions

1. Place chopped onions and peppers into a large soup pot or dutch oven. Sauté in a little veggie broth until translucent and softened.
2. Add minced garlic and sauté for an additional 30 seconds until fragrant.
3. Add any kind of meat substitute (if using) or dry, uncooked bulgur and continue to stir for a few minutes until heated through.
4. Add tomatoes, tomato sauce, and remaining broth Add in spices and stir until mixed well
5. Add all the beans and jalapeños and stir.
6. Give the chili one more good stir and bring it to a slow boil. Reduce heat, cover, and simmer for 15 to 30 minutes.
7. Serve with the Garlic Turmeric Rice and Sliced Avocado
8. *It gets better every day it chills in the refrigerator and the flavors meld together*

Veggie Soup (Not Chicken)

This "Not Chicken" Veggie Soup marries tradition with modernity, giving a plant-based nod to classic chicken soup. Crafted with avocado oil, onions, carrots, celery, garlic, and vegan "no chicken" bouillon, this recipe draws on the indigenous practice of using local, natural ingredients for nourishment. It reflects contemporary shifts towards healthier, sustainable diets without sacrificing the comfort of a timeless soup. With optional noodles for added heartiness, "Not Chicken" Veggie Soup is a culinary celebration of America's diverse heritage, inviting everyone to enjoy a dish that's both inclusive and deliciously comforting.

Ingredients

- ¼ Cup Avocado Oil
- 2 Medium Yellow Onion
- 6 Carrots
- 3 Stalks Celery
- 6 Cloves Garlic
- 8 Cups Water
- 4 Cubes Vegan No Chicken Bouillon 3 Bay Leaves
- Salt and Pepper to taste 8 Oz Noodles *Optional*

Instructions

1. In a large soup pot, heat oil on medium heat. Add in the carrots, celery, and onion. Sauté until carrots are tender, about 5 minutes.
2. Mix in the garlic and cook for another minute.
3. Add in the water, bouillon, bay leaves, pepper, and salt. Bring to a simmer on medium-high.
4. Add in the noodles. Cook until noodles are al dente (this will depend on the type of noodle you choose - check the package for cooking time.)

Nutrition Facts

Serving size: 1 Cup
Servings: 10

Amount per serving

Calories   564

% Daily Value*

Total Fat 7g	9%
Saturated Fat 2.3g	11%
Cholesterol 0mg	0%
Sodium 738mg	32%
Total Carbohydrate 111.3g	40%
Dietary Fiber 22.8g	82%
Total Sugars 7.7g	
Protein 22.3g	
Vitamin D 0mcg	0%
Calcium 470mg	36%
Iron 21mg	116%
Potassium 1176mg	25%

*The % Daily Value (DV) tells you how much a nutrient in a food serving contributes to a daily diet. 2,000 calorie a day is used for general nutrition advice.

Recipe analyzed by verywell

Ch 2: Soups + Sauces : Veggie Soup

Brown Sauce (Manchurian)

Brown Sauce (Manchurian) is the epitome of a vibrant testament to culinary fusion. It marries together century-old traditional Asian flavors with the spirit of American innovation. This recipe has ginger, garlic, soy sauce, and vegan fish sauce and umami instead of classic Manchurian sauce. Its preparation embodies the principle of Native Americans in respect and harmony with the gifts of nature. It gives us food both insipid on a global scale and deeply rooted in sustainable eating practice. This sauce invites an international audience to explore a tapestry of flavors that bridges continents and cultures on a shared plate.

Ingredients

- 2 Tbsp Neutral Cooking Oil
- 2 Tbsp Ginger (minced)
- 2 Tbsp Garlic (minced)
- 1/2 Cup Veggie Broth
- 2 Tbsp Sesame Oil
- 1/4 Cup Dark Soy Sauce
- 1/3 Cup Light Soy Sauce
- 1/4 Cup Vegan Fish Sauce
- 1 Tbsp Vegan Umami
- 1/4 Cup Rice Wine Vinegar
- 1/3 Cup Mirin (Optional)
- 1 Tsp White Pepper
- 1 Tsp Onion Power
- 1 Tsp Garlic Powder
- 1/4 Cup Brown Sugar

* Optional Thickener *
- 1 Tbsp Chickpea Flour
- 2 Tbsp Spring Water

Nutrition Facts

Serving size: 2 Tablespoons
Servings: 12

Amount per serving
Calories 235

	% Daily Value*
Total Fat 17.8g	23%
Saturated Fat 2.6g	13%
Cholesterol 0mg	0%
Sodium 757mg	33%
Total Carbohydrate 19.1g	7%
Dietary Fiber 3.4g	12%
Total Sugars 7.6g	
Protein 2.6g	
Vitamin D 0mcg	0%
Calcium 52mg	4%
Iron 3mg	15%
Potassium 201mg	4%

The % Daily Value (DV) tells you how much a nutrient in a food serving contributes to a daily diet. 2,000 calorie a day is used for general nutrition advice.

Recipe analyzed by well

Instructions

1. Premix ingredients in a bowl, cook on medium heat until thickened.
2. Let cool and store in an airtight jar to use anytime.

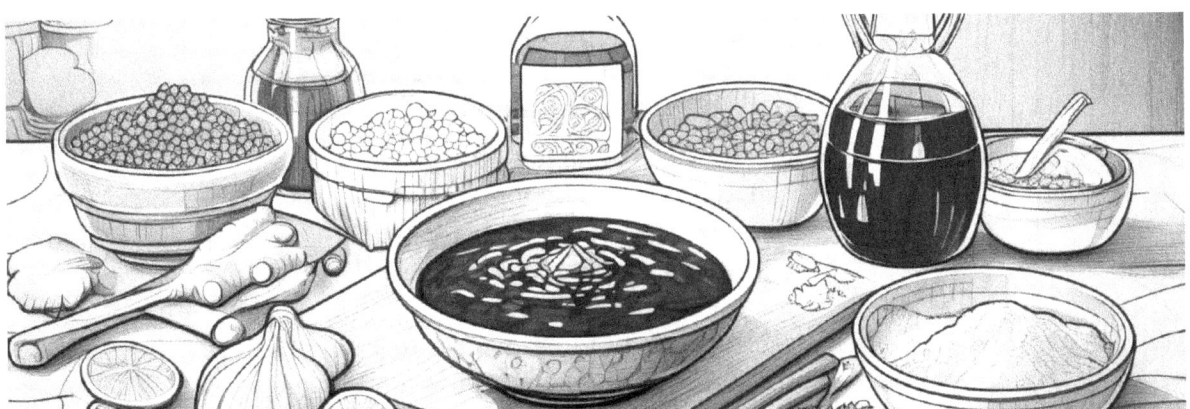

Ch 2: Soups + Sauces : Brown Sauce

Red Sauce

Red Sauce redefines simplicity and versatility in the kitchen. From starting with your favorite brand out of a jar, like Raos, to crafting it yourself from fresh or canned Roma tomatoes, this recipe is certain to bring forth the ultimate flavor. A rainbow of bell peppers, zucchini, and a hearty, robust blend of roasted garlic, garlic powder, onion powder, and Italian seasoning—all sautéed in avocado oil—give a home to the otherwise modest tomato base, transforming it into a rich, aromatic sauce. Perfect for your pasta, pizza, or even dipping, the red sauce invites one to serve and savor the taste of home, much like the one you grew up with and loved.

Ingredients

- 1 Can Peeled Roma Tomatoes (Diced Roma Tomatoes or your favorite jar of sauce can work well too)
- 1 Large Yellow Onion
- 5 Cloves Roasted Garlic
- 1 Green Pepper
- 1 Red Pepper
- 1 Yellow Pepper
- 1 Orange Pepper
- 1 Zucchini
- 3 Tbsp Avocado Oil
- 3 Tbsp Garlic Powder
- 3 Tbsp Onion Powder
- 4 Tbsp Italian Seasoning

Instructions

1. Heat avocado oil in a sauce pan. Add onions to sauté until they're translucent.
2. Add garlic and mix through.
3. Add a mix of bell peppers (red, green, yellow, orange, perhaps zucchini) to the garlic/ onion mix
4. Start to season by adding a blend of fresh or dried herbs consisting of basil, rosemary, thyme, oregano, marjoram and sage, pink Himalayan sea salt and pepper to taste.
5. Lastly, add the canned tomatoes to the pan, stir well and simmer.

Optional

- Add cooked pasta with a few tablespoons of pasta water for a traditional pasta dish or completely cool and store in an airtight jar.
- Fresh diced Roma tomatoes, canned diced Roma tomatoes or tomato sauce can be substituted with great success; if using fresh tomatoes adding a couple of tablespoons of tomato paste to lift the flavor can be beneficial.

Nutrition Facts

Serving size: 1/8 Cup
Servings: 8

Amount per serving
Calories 616

	% Daily Value*
Total Fat 22.8g	29%
Saturated Fat 4g	20%
Cholesterol 34mg	11%
Sodium 270mg	12%
Total Carbohydrate 97.2g	35%
Dietary Fiber 12.2g	44%
Total Sugars 33.2g	
Protein 16.9g	
Vitamin D 0mcg	0%
Calcium 340mg	26%
Iron 5mg	30%
Potassium 1618mg	34%

*The % Daily Value (DV) tells you how much a nutrient in a food serving contributes to a daily diet. 2,000 calorie a day is used for general nutrition advice.

Recipe analyzed by verywell

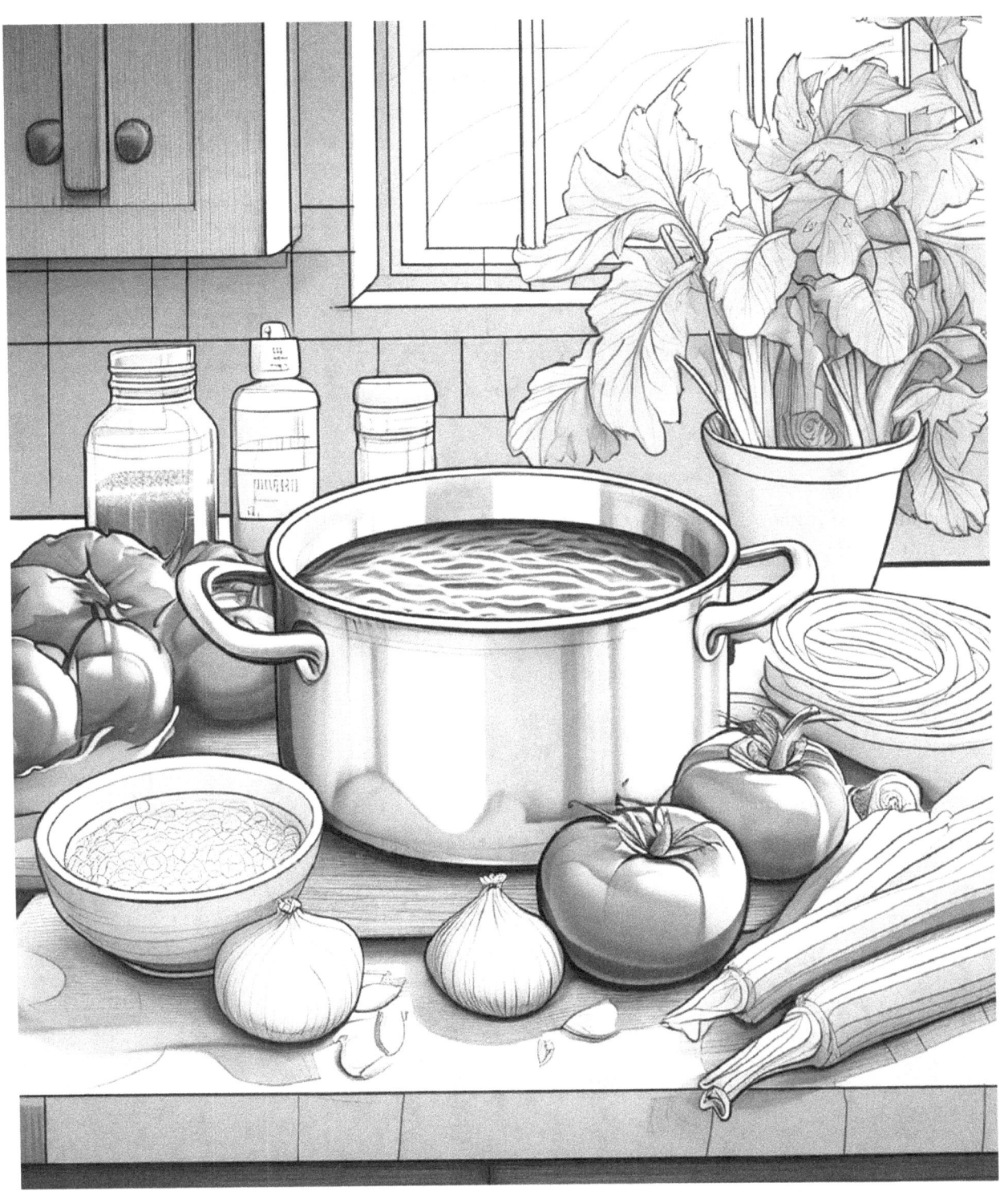

Ch 2: Soups + Sauces : Red Sauce

Creamy Alfredo Sauce

Perfectly creamy, vegan Alfredo sauce is not from a jar; it is homemade for a rich, authentic flavor, just like the traditional non-vegan versions. The secret is to replace the parmesan with something intriguing that hemp seeds have to offer to get that plant-based creaminess. That, with a splash of water, loads of roasted garlic for an extra flavor hit, onion powder, and a mix of Italian herbs. "This recipe takes classic and turns it vegan without losing the taste or texture—it's not just an imitation of the original Alfredo but holds its own.

Ingredients

- 2 cups Hemp Seed
- 2 cups Spring Water
- 1/3 cup Garlic Powder (*Roasted will add an amazing touch)
- 1/3 cup Onion Powder
- 1/4 cup Italian Herbal Blend (Basil, Oregano, Marjoram, Thyme, Savory, Rosemary, Sage,)
- Salt and Pepper to taste

Instructions

- Add all ingredients to blender, blend on high until smooth then add directly to cooked pasta or store in an airtight jar.

Nutrition Facts

Serving size: 1/8 Cup
Servings: 8

Amount per serving

Calories 178

	% Daily Value*
Total Fat 10.1g	13%
Saturated Fat 1.7g	8%
Cholesterol 0mg	0%
Sodium 3mg	0%
Total Carbohydrate 11.4g	4%
Dietary Fiber 4g	14%
Total Sugars 2.5g	
Protein 9.5g	
Vitamin D 0mcg	0%
Calcium 18mg	1%
Iron 2mg	11%
Potassium 85mg	2%

*The % Daily Value (DV) tells you how much a nutrient in a food serving contributes to a daily diet. 2,000 calorie a day is used for general nutrition advice.

Recipe analyzed by verywell

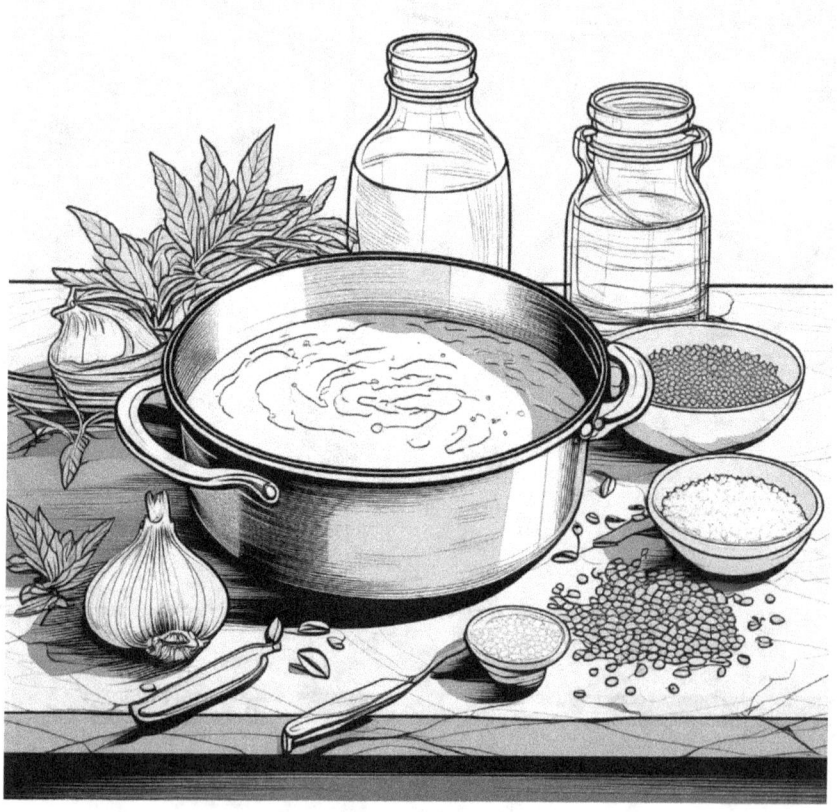

Ch 2: Soups + Sauces : Alfredo

Pesto

Pesto gets the vegan treatment in this fun take. Made usually with basil, pine nuts, and Parmesan, this includes walnuts and hemp seeds, swapping in for pine nuts and keeping the cheese out. But it still maintains that vibrant, herby essence of classic pesto while adding in a unique nuttiness complexity. Fresh basil is the dominant flavor, mixing with pungent garlic and rich extra virgin olive oil to give the sauce something between familiar and novelty. This is a flexible, inventive take on pesto; a plant-based alternative to drizzle over pastas, sandwiches, or salads; something for any kind of eater to enjoy.

Ingredients

- 4 Cups Fresh Basil
- 1/4 Cup Walnuts
- 5 Cloves Garlic
- 1/4 Cup Hemp Seeds
- 1/3 Cup Extra Virgin Olive Oil
- Salt and Pepper to Taste

Instructions

1. Add all ingredients to a food processor. Process on low checking the consistency.
2. Add directly to cooked pasta (hot or cold) or store in an airtight jar.

Nutrition Facts

Serving size: 1/8 Cup
Servings: 8

Amount per serving

Calories   176

% Daily Value*

Total Fat 7.6g	10%
Saturated Fat 1g	5%
Cholesterol 0mg	0%
Sodium 13mg	1%
Total Carbohydrate 22.9g	8%
Dietary Fiber 2.7g	10%
Total Sugars 0.8g	
Protein 7.4g	
Vitamin D 0mcg	0%
Calcium 204mg	16%
Iron 3mg	17%
Potassium 415mg	9%

*The % Daily Value (DV) tells you how much a nutrient in a food serving contributes to a daily diet. 2,000 calorie a day is used for general nutrition advice.

Recipe analyzed by **well**

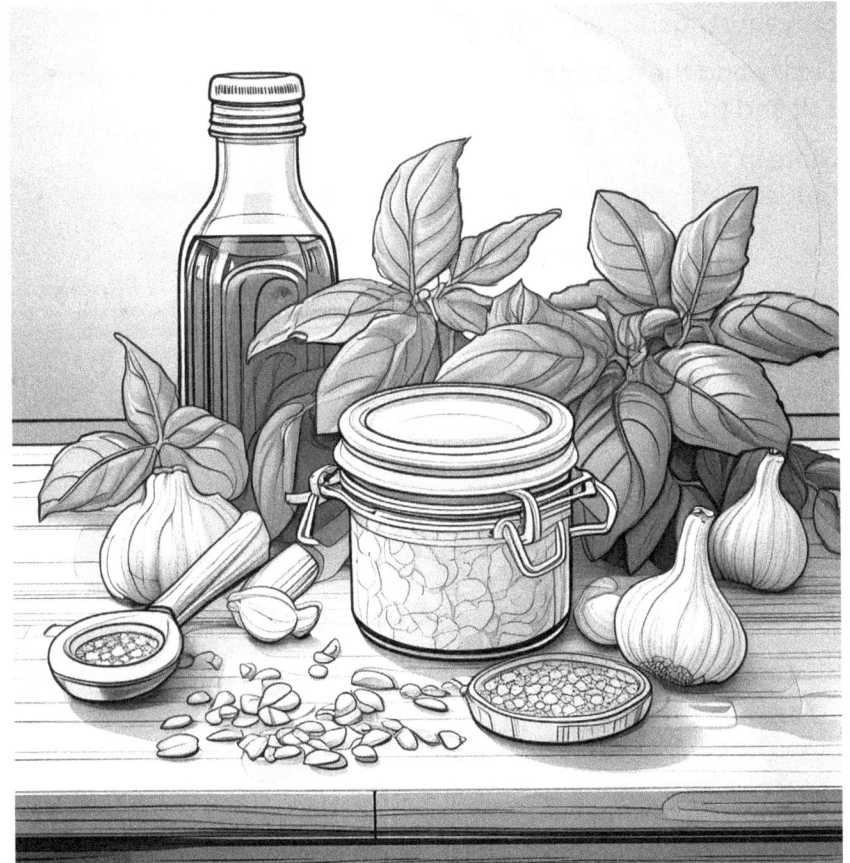

Ch 2: Soups + Sauces : Pesto

Tzatziki

This vegan tzatziki recipe gives the beloved Mediterranean condiment a refreshing makeover. We keep the creamy texture and tangy taste of classic tzatziki using either unsweetened plain vegan yogurt or vegan mayo, hence retaining the soul of this classic sauce but at the same time making it available to all. Freshly grated cucumber, aromatic garlic, bright dill, and a perfectly mixed amount of black pepper and sea salt all humbly combined to create a harmonious mixture that was invigorating yet comfortingly known. This vegan rendition proves that classic recipes are easily open to modern dietary preferences by using a plant-based counterpart to all sorts of dishes.

Ingredients

- 1 Tbsp Garlic
- 1 Tsp Black Pepper
- 1 Tsp Sea Salt
- 1 Cucumber
- 1/2 cup Fresh Dill
- 1/2 cup Vegan Mayo (Unsweetened Plain Vegan Yogurt)

Instructions

1. Start by placing a clean kitchen towel into a bowl. Grate cucumber into the bowl then lightly sprinkle with sea salt to draw out the water.
2. Pull towel together and wring out as much of the excess water as possible. Drink or set aside for later use.
3. In a separate bowl add mayonnaise (or yogurt) garlic, and dill.
4. Finally add the cucumber, mix well, salt and pepper to taste.
5. Store in a airtight jar or squeeze bottle.

Nutrition Facts

Serving size: 2 Tablespoons
Servings: 4

Amount per serving

Calories 129

	% Daily Value*
Total Fat 9.6g	12%
Saturated Fat 1g	5%
Cholesterol 0mg	0%
Sodium 217mg	9%
Total Carbohydrate 11g	4%
Dietary Fiber 2.3g	8%
Total Sugars 1.3g	
Protein 3.2g	
Vitamin D 0mcg	0%
Calcium 242mg	19%
Iron 7mg	36%
Potassium 542mg	12%

*The % Daily Value (DV) tells you how much a nutrient in a food serving contributes to a daily diet. 2,000 calorie a day is used for general nutrition advice.

Recipe analyzed by verywell

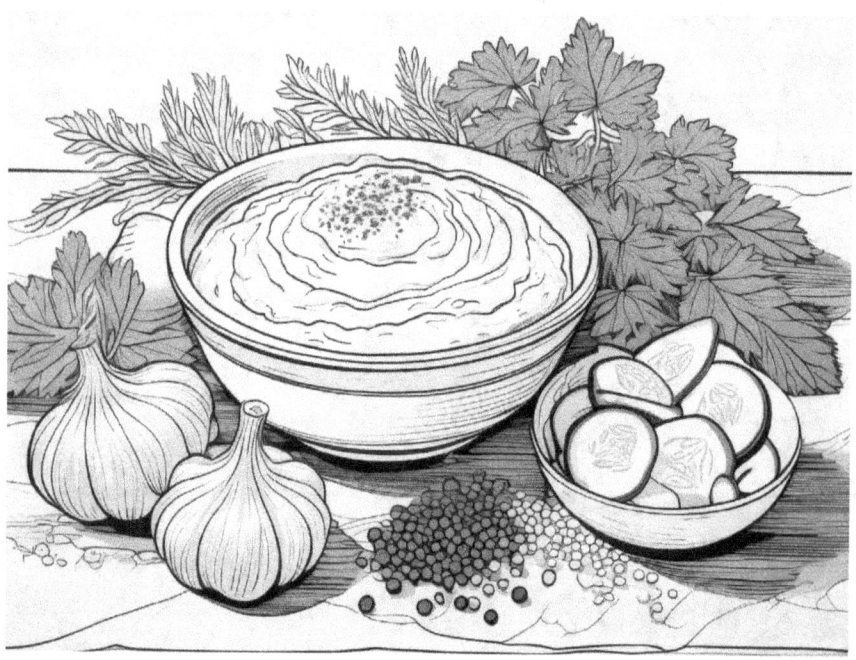

Garlic Tahini

Tahini Garlic Sauce is one of the simple and multi-tasking recipes in vegan cuisines. It can be used in blending art; as a matter of fact, by gradually mixing in the liquid, the tahini finally turns out into a creamy, pourable dressing. Add fresh lemon or tangy key lime juice for that perfect acid balance. Water the sauce to get the right consistency. Add roasted or powdered garlic for that full-flavored garlic taste. Add a pinch of sea salt to taste. Emulsify. But this garlic tahini is no ordinary condiment. It's an excellent explosion of flavor that takes everything up to their limits, showing the power of just simple ingredients, artfully combined.

Ingredients

- ½ Cup Tahini
- ¼ Cup Fresh Lemon Juice (2 - 4 Tbsp Key Lime Juice can be substituted)
- 6 Tbsp water, plus more as needed
- 3 Cloves Garlic (Roasted Minced Garlic or fine garlic powder can be a good substitute)
- ½ Tsp Sea Salt

Instructions

1. Tahini sauces are super easy and really come down to technique. By slowly mixing the liquids with the tahini you will notice the consistency of the tahini changes to more of a sauce.

2. Adding your favorite spices and or herbs (garlic in this case) you will have a flavorful sauce that you can put on a lot of different dishes.

Nutrition Facts

Serving size: 2 Tablespoons
Servings: 16

Amount per serving

Calories   **20**

% Daily Value*

Total Fat 1.7g	2%
Saturated Fat 0.3g	1%
Cholesterol 0mg	0%
Sodium 21mg	1%
Total Carbohydrate 0.9g	0%
Dietary Fiber 0.3g	1%
Total Sugars 0.1g	
Protein 0.6g	
Vitamin D 0mcg	0%
Calcium 16mg	1%
Iron 0mg	2%
Potassium 20mg	0%

*The % Daily Value (DV) tells you how much a nutrient in a food serving contributes to a daily diet. 2,000 calorie a day is used for general nutrition advice.

Recipe analyzed by **well**

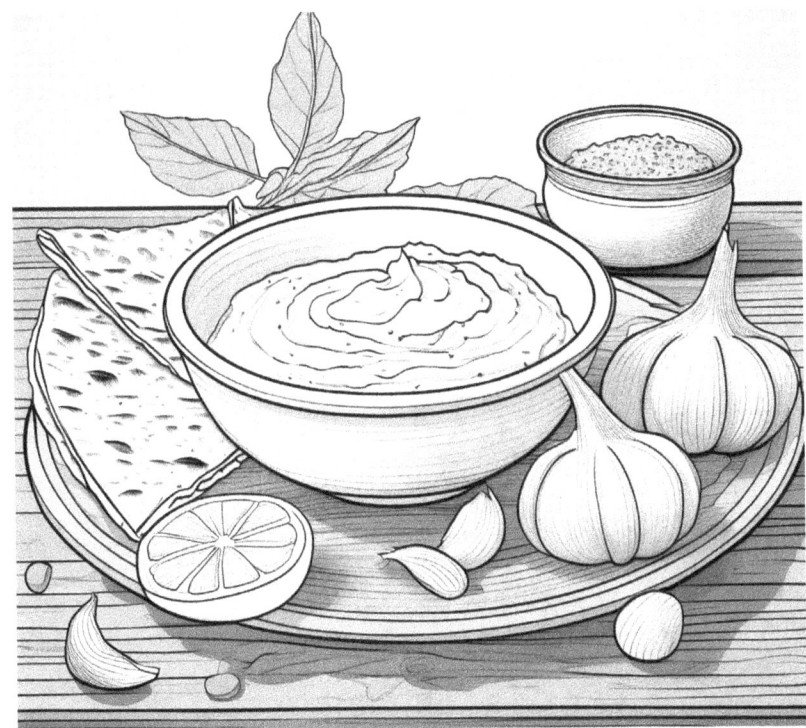

Guacamole

Guacamole—that all-time favorite. It brings together ripe avocados, Roma tomatoes, crispy yellow onion, and pungent garlic, with the zesty accent of key lime, all seasoned with salt and pepper. This recipe certainly celebrates the rich, creamy texture of an avocado—staple to the cuisines of indigenous America—letting each ingredient play a part in raising those natural flavors. The key lime offers that citrus note, breaking through the richness and giving just a beautiful taste profile. It's more than a dip or spread—it's the culinary expression of tradition and simplicity in every bowl. It provides an excuse for any dish to be enjoyed in countless ways, from many regions, all connecting at the table.

Ingredients

- 4 Avocados
- 2 Roma Tomatoes
- 1/2 Large Yellow Onion
- 3 Cloves Garlic
- 1 Key Lime
- Salt and Pepper to taste

Instructions

1. Start by cubing the avocados and dicing the tomatoes, then the onions.
2. Mince garlic and cut the key lime.
3. In a large bowl add two avocados and lightly smash. Then add tomatoes, onions and garlic. Gently mix.
4. Add the other two avocados squeeze the juice of the key lime and gently mix.
5. Salt and pepper to taste.

Nutrition Facts

Serving size: 1/2 Cup
Servings: 4

Amount per serving
Calories 449

	% Daily Value*
Total Fat 39.5g	51%
Saturated Fat 8.3g	41%
Cholesterol 0mg	0%
Sodium 19mg	1%
Total Carbohydrate 26.6g	10%
Dietary Fiber 15.6g	56%
Total Sugars 4.6g	
Protein 5.4g	
Vitamin D 0mcg	0%
Calcium 55mg	4%
Iron 2mg	10%
Potassium 1262mg	27%

*The % Daily Value (DV) tells you how much a nutrient in a food serving contributes to a daily diet. 2,000 calorie a day is used for general nutrition advice.

Recipe analyzed by verywell

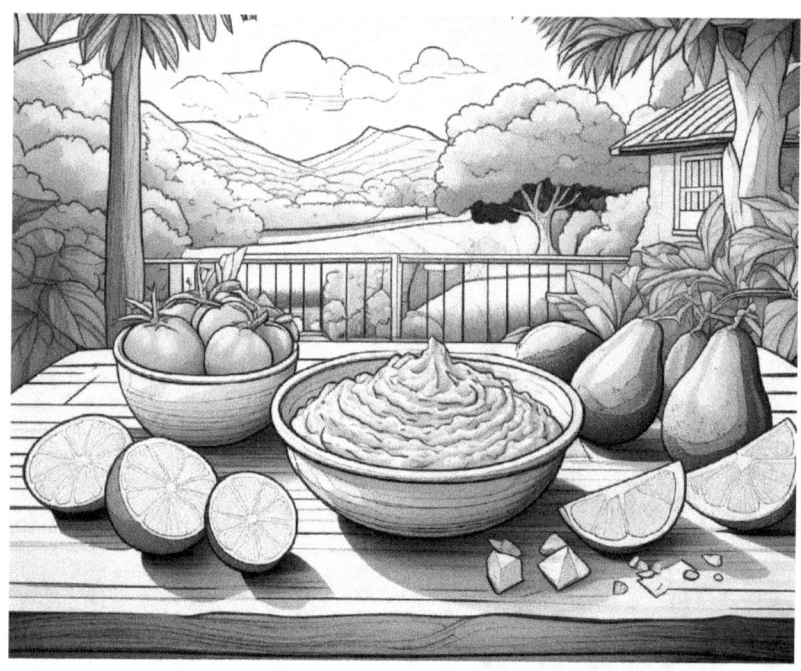

Salsa (Pico de Gallo)

Pico de Gallo is an energetic, colorful mix: fresh, diced Roma tomatoes combine with crisp red onion and hot Serrano or jalapeño peppers. All of this is perked up with a squeeze of key lime juice. Further enriched with the fresh, aromatic presence of cilantro, seasoned with oregano and cumin for depth, this recipe is not concocting a condiment—it is personifying the spirit of freshness and flavor, offering a taste of a rich culinary heritage. And every one of them plays a truly central role, contributing every one of its bold, refreshing tastes. Perfect as a condiment or all-purpose side, Pico de Gallo finds a way to bridge the past and the present, bringing the essence of traditional flavors to your diverse table today.

Ingredients

- 4 - 6 Roma Tomatoes (1 to 1 1/2 pounds)
- 1/2 Red Onion
- 2 Serrano or 1 jalapeño Pepper (less or more to taste)
- Juice of 1 Key Lime
- 1/2 Cup Cilantro
- 1 Tbsp Oregano
- 1 Tsp Cumin

Instructions

1. Start by dicing tomatoes, onion and peppers.
2. Add to a large bowl with seasonings and gently mix.
3. Finish with squeezing the juice of the key lime, mix well.
4. Store in an airtight jar.

Nutrition Facts

Serving size: 1/2 Cup
Servings: 6

Amount per serving

Calories   143

% Daily Value*

Total Fat 5.7g	7%
Saturated Fat 0.7g	4%
Cholesterol 0mg	0%
Sodium 41mg	2%
Total Carbohydrate 25.1g	9%
Dietary Fiber 11.1g	39%
Total Sugars 4.5g	
Protein 6.3g	
Vitamin D 0mcg	0%
Calcium 440mg	34%
Iron 19mg	105%
Potassium 918mg	20%

*The % Daily Value (DV) tells you how much a nutrient in a food serving contributes to a daily diet. 2,000 calorie a day is used for general nutrition advice.

Recipe analyzed by **well**

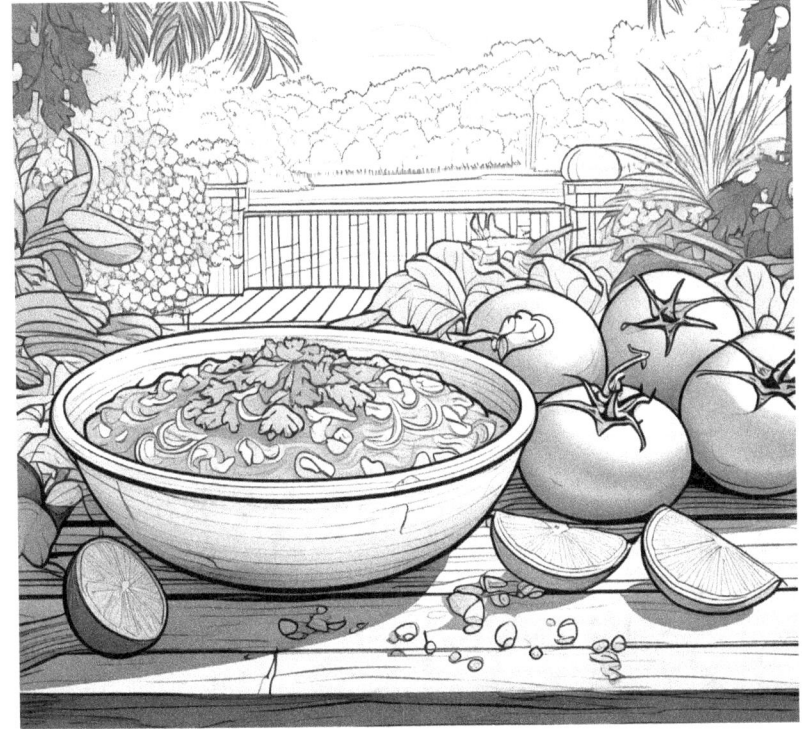

Ch 2: Soups + Sauces : Salsa

Jerk Sauce (Marinade)

Jerk Sauce is a flavor-bursting marinade that is the cornerstone of Caribbean cuisine, representing deep fusion in culinary arts and the influences of spice trading. Fresh scallions, thyme, and optional celery, or broad-leaf thyme, combine with pungent garlic, warm ginger, and the aromatic kick of allspice and pimento peppers. Scotch bonnet peppers bring in their recognizably hot taste, while chopped onions, salt, black pepper, and grated nutmeg all add to a complexity of flavor. Browning adds depth and color, sugar tones down the heat, and vegetable oil brings everything together. A final splash of vinegar and citrus juice rounds out this hot, rich, versatile jerk sauce that will bring the authentic, lively Caribbean tradition into your cooking.

Ingredients

- Fresh Scallion and Thyme
- Celery leaves or Broad Leaf Thyme (optional)
- Garlic Cloves (4-5 pieces)
- Ginger 3-4 Small Slices
- 1 Tbsp Pimento Seeds (All Spice Berries)
- 4-5 Pimento Peppers (For Flavor) if Available
- 1 Scotch Bonnet Pepper, More for More Spice
- 1 Onion (Chopped)
- 1 Tsp Salt
- 1/2 Tsp Black Pepper
- 1/2 Tsp Grated Nutmeg
- 1-2 Tbsp Browning
- 1 Tbsp Sugar
- 1 Tbsp Vegetable Oil
- White Vinegar
- Slash of Lime and/or Lemon Juice (Sour Orange if Available)

Nutrition Facts

Serving size: 1/2 Cup
Servings: 4

Amount per serving
Calories 195

	% Daily Value*
Total Fat 1.1g	1%
Saturated Fat 0.3g	2%
Cholesterol 0mg	0%
Sodium 18mg	1%
Total Carbohydrate 48.8g	18%
Dietary Fiber 8.6g	31%
Total Sugars 28g	
Protein 4.5g	
Vitamin D 0mcg	0%
Calcium 205mg	16%
Iron 9mg	49%
Potassium 506mg	11%

*The % Daily Value (DV) tells you how much a nutrient in a food serving contributes to a daily diet. 2,000 calorie a day is used for general nutrition advice.

Recipe analyzed by verywell

Instructions

1. Add all ingredients to food processor and blitz until combined.
2. Store in an airtight jar.
3. Use to marinate vegetables or add agave to make one of the best jerk sauces ever.

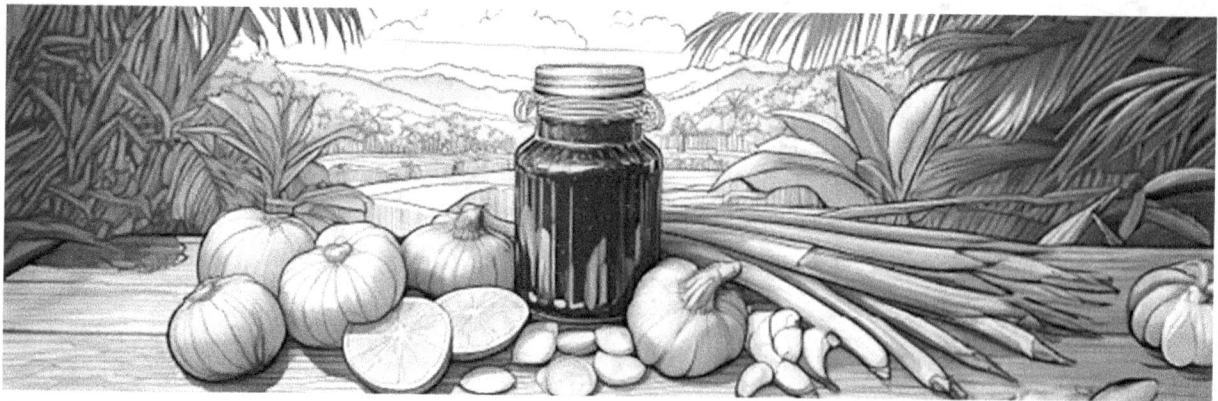

Ch 2: Soups + Sauces : Jerk Sauce

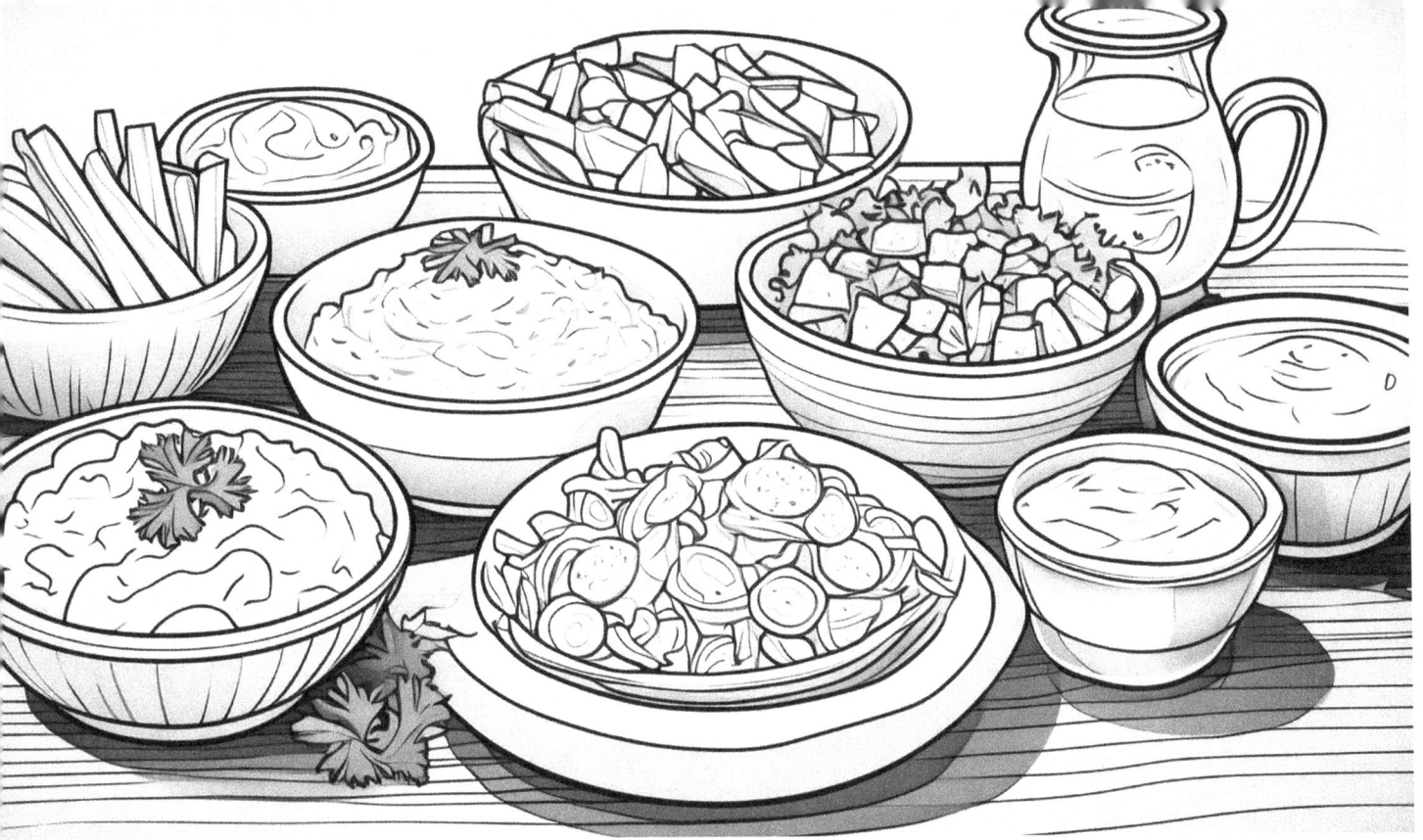

3.
SIDES
[AND]
STARTERS

This chapter explores a variety of delectable side dishes and starters to complement any vegan meal. From creamy hummus and flavorful dressings to fresh slaws and veggie sautés, these recipes showcase the incredible versatility of plant-based ingredients. Start with the tantalizing pasta or potato salad dressing that combines rich vegan mayo, zesty mustard, and vibrant relish. The kale and cabbage slaw is a crisp and refreshing addition bursting with colors and textures. For a protein-packed starter, the classic hummus provides a dreamy base to customize with your favorite flavors. The simple house dressing is an all-purpose vinaigrette imbued with Italian seasonings. Explore unique dishes like the wakame seaweed salad inspired by Japanese cuisine. Complete your meal with quick veggie sautés that allow the natural flavors of seasonal produce to shine. With this array of sides and starters, you'll have plenty of delicious options to elevate your vegan dining experience.

Pasta / Potato Salad Dressing

This Pasta/Potato Salad Dressing brings the tangy bite of yellow mustard together with creamy vegan mayo to marry two potent, rich bases into one harmonious whole. Sweet relish adds a hint of both sweetness and complexity, while the onion comes in crisp and savory. Flavor every bite with the goodness of garlic and onion powders, let it round with dashes of salt and pepper. But taste is not all that will bring you back to this dressing. It's perfect for dressing pasta salads, topping off potato salads, or drizzling over your favorite salad greens as a simple and tasty way to add a kick to any meal. With an appeal as wide as mass appeal and staying true to plant-based diets, this dressing always delivers.

Ingredients

- 1/2 Cup Vegan Mayo
- 1/2 Cup Yellow Mustard
- 1/3 Cup Sweet Relish
- 1/2 Diced Onion
- 1 Tbsp Garlic Powder
- 1 Tbsp Onion Powder
- Salt and Pepper to taste

Instructions

For Pasta Salad:

1. In a large bowl mix all ingredients.
2. Boil pasta of choice according to instructions. Rinse with cold water then add to the large bowl with the mix.
3. Mix well until everything is coated then refrigerate.

For Potato Salad:

1. Wash and cube potatoes, then add cubed potatoes to a pot of boiling water.
2. While potatoes cook, mix all other ingredients in a bowl.
3. When potatoes are tender, strain and quickly rinse under cold water.
4. Allow potatoes to completely cool. Once cooled, add potatoes to the bowl with mixture.
5. Mix well until potatoes are fully coated then refrigerate.

Nutrition Facts

Servings: 8

Amount per serving

Calories 61

	% Daily Value*
Total Fat 4.5g	6%
Saturated Fat 0.5g	2%
Cholesterol 0mg	0%
Sodium 194mg	8%
Total Carbohydrate 5.3g	2%
Dietary Fiber 0.3g	1%
Total Sugars 3.6g	
Protein 0.3g	
Vitamin D 0mcg	0%
Calcium 5mg	0%
Iron 0mg	1%
Potassium 26mg	1%

*The % Daily Value (DV) tells you how much a nutrient in a food serving contributes to a daily diet. 2,000 calorie a day is used for general nutrition advice.

Recipe analyzed by verywell

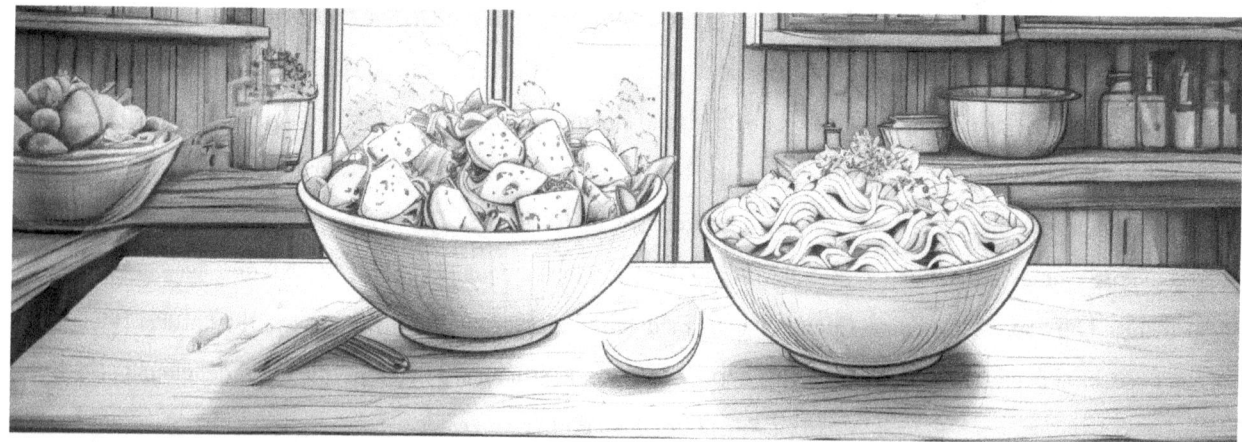

Slaw

This reinterpretation of the classic slaw salad combines kale with cabbage and broccoli for a light and fresh base. The dressing strikes a perfect balance between sweet and acidic from the creamy vegan mayonnaise and tang of apple cider vinegar, respectively, then lightly sweetened by drizzling in some agave. It is well seasoned with salt and a healthy dose of pepper if you like a peppery bite, but this slaw is more than just a side—it really is one of those things that make a meal a meal. An excellent pick for the health-conscious diner looking to place a pop of both taste and color onto his plate, embodying a new look at an old favorite, slaw.

Ingredients

- 1 cup ea of kale, cabbage, broccoli

Dressing

- 1/2 cup vegan mayo
- 1/4 cup vinegar / apple cider vinegar 1/8 cup agave
- salt + pepper to taste (I like peppery slaw)

Instructions

Whisk ingredients until smooth then add to your shredded veggies.

This recipe is super simple and a necessary addition to BBQ Shredded Jackfruit sandwiches.

Nutrition Facts

Servings: 8

Amount per serving

Calories   45

% Daily Value*

Total Fat 4.5g	6%
Saturated Fat 0.5g	2%
Cholesterol 0mg	0%
Sodium 36mg	2%
Total Carbohydrate 1.2g	0%
Dietary Fiber 0.1g	0%
Total Sugars 1.1g	
Protein 0g	
Vitamin D 0mcg	0%
Calcium 0mg	0%
Iron 0mg	0%
Potassium 0mg	0%

*The % Daily Value (DV) tells you how much a nutrient in a food serving contributes to a daily diet. 2,000 calorie a day is used for general nutrition advice.

Recipe analyzed by **well**

Hummus

Hummus is the base dish for this; it's a palate of culinary creativity. It's not more than a simple base with pureed chickpeas, aquafaba, and tahini; the rest is complemented with olive oil. Some might add a squeeze of lemon, and if that's their choice, so be it, but never would the author desecrate such a delicious taste with minced garlic, roasted red peppers, or everything seasoning. With that in mind, this approach to hummus is therefore about celebrating personal preference, allowing each batch to take shape as a reflection of one's individual taste but always with the creamy, satisfying essence that makes this Middle Eastern spread so beloved.

Ingredients

- 1 can chickpeas (garbanzo beans)
- 1/4 cup aquafaba
- 1/4 cup tahini
- 2 tablespoons olive oil
- salt and pepper to taste

Instructions

1. Process tahini and lemon juice in a food processor for 1 minute, scraping sides.
2. Add olive oil, garlic, cumin (optional), and salt. Process 30 seconds, scrape, then process again until blended.
3. Pulse in half the chickpeas, scrape, then add remaining and process 1-2 minutes for a thick and creamy texture.
4. Gradually add aquafaba while processing until desired consistency is reached.
5. Taste and adjust seasonings. Serve with pita bread, veggies, or crackers.

Nutrition Facts

Servings: 6

Amount per serving

Calories 352

	% Daily Value*
Total Fat 34.4g	44%
Saturated Fat 4.9g	24%
Cholesterol 0mg	0%
Sodium 9mg	0%
Total Carbohydrate 11g	4%
Dietary Fiber 3.3g	12%
Total Sugars 1.8g	
Protein 3.9g	
Vitamin D 0mcg	0%
Calcium 35mg	3%
Iron 1mg	8%
Potassium 163mg	3%

*The % Daily Value (DV) tells you how much a nutrient in a food serving contributes to a daily diet. 2,000 calorie a day is used for general nutrition advice.

Recipe analyzed by verywell

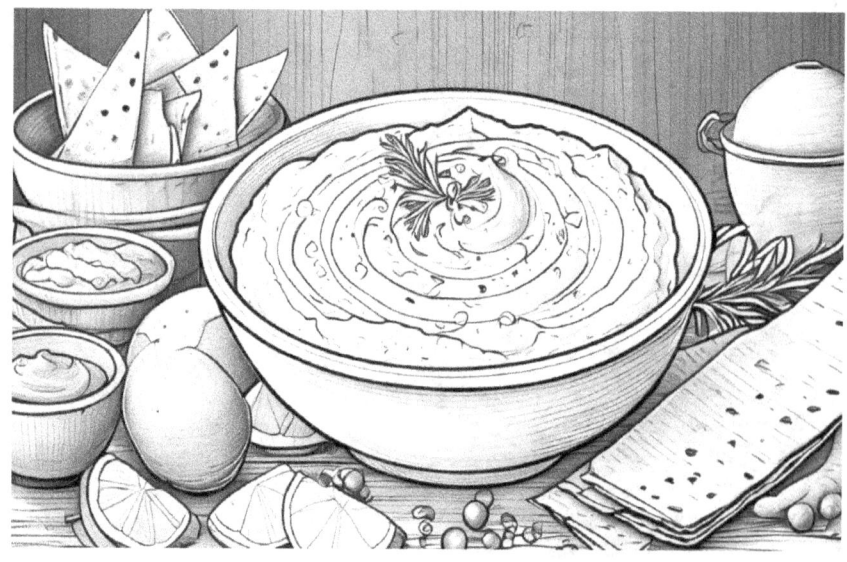

Simple House Dressing

Simple House Dressing epitomizes the charm of uncomplicated yet flavorful preparations. A quick fix for year-round salad dressing, this marries olive oil with apple cider vinegar to just the right suggestion of richness and tang. A hint of agave brings just the right amount of sweetness to round out the flavors, while a combination of Italian seasonings introduces fragrant herbs that introduce a completely new take on the dressing. Season with appropriate amount of salt and pepper, this is generally the all-rounder, adaptable dressing that enhances not only the salads but the veggie dish as well. The salad is made in minutes and, conveniently, it stores in the fridge to add a fresh, homemade flair to meals over the week.

Ingredients

- 1/4 cup Olive Oil
- 1/4 cup Apple Cider Vinegar
- 1 tsp Agave
- Italian Seasoning Blend
- Salt and Pepper to taste

Instructions

Mix all ingredients in a bottle, shake and enjoy.

Make sure to shake well after refrigerating.

Nutrition Facts

Serving size: 1 tablespoon
Servings: 6

Amount per serving

Calories 125

% Daily Value*

Total Fat 4.4g	6%
Saturated Fat 0.7g	4%
Cholesterol 0mg	0%
Sodium 8mg	0%
Total Carbohydrate 23.5g	9%
Dietary Fiber 5.2g	19%
Total Sugars 12g	
Protein 1.8g	
Vitamin D 0mcg	0%
Calcium 74mg	6%
Iron 5mg	27%
Potassium 213mg	5%

*The % Daily Value (DV) tells you how much a nutrient in a food serving contributes to a daily diet. 2,000 calorie a day is used for general nutrition advice.

Recipe analyzed by **well**

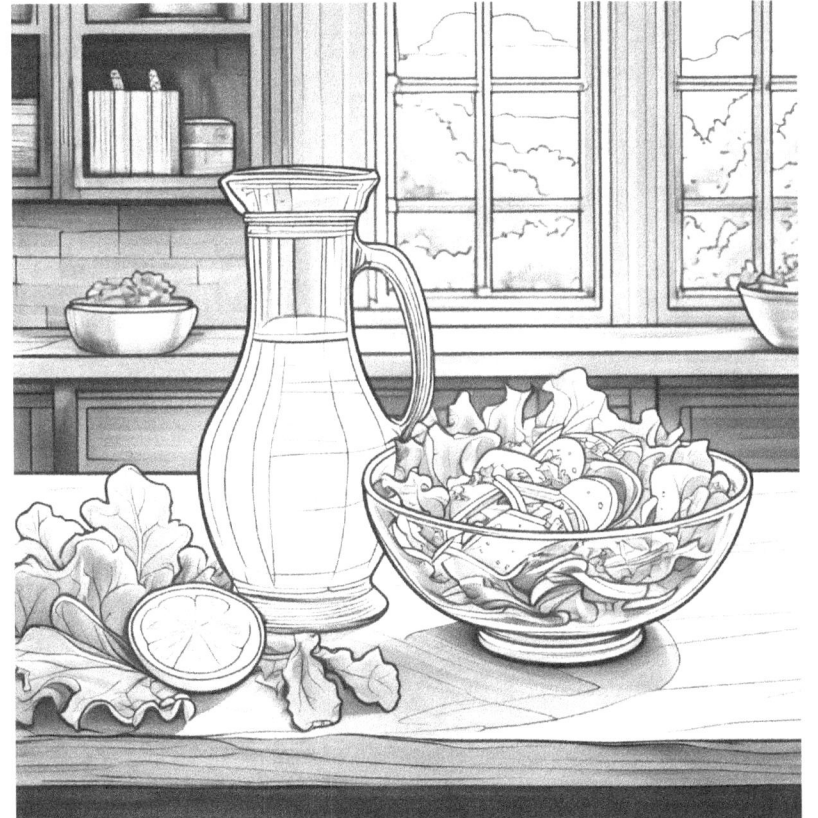

Ch 2: Soups + Sauces : Dressing

Seaweed Salad (Wakame)

Made of seaweed, Wakame Salad is very simple but at the same time, a very sophisticated mixture of textures and flavors, traditional for Japanese cuisine. Soaked dried wakame is combined here with savory reduced-sodium soy sauce and tangy rice vinegar. Optional mirin adds sweetness, while grated ginger and garlic bring warmth and zest. To give it richness, add in the toasted sesame oil and a little nutty heat from the red pepper flakes. For an added touch of freshness, you can add thinly sliced baby cucumbers in the mix along with the toasted white sesame seeds for an incredible crunch. This is an unabashed salad celebration of seaweed's versatility, flavor, and balance.

Ingredients

- 1 Tbsp dried wakame seaweed
- 3 tablespoons reduced-sodium soy sauce 1 tablespoon rice vinegar
- 1 tablespoon mirin *OPTIONAL* 1 teaspoon sugar
- 1 teaspoon grated ginger
- ½ teaspoon grated garlic
- 1 tablespoon toasted sesame oil
- ¼ teaspoon red pepper flakes
- 1 baby cucumber (skin on), very thinly sliced
- ½ teaspoon toasted white sesame seeds

Instructions

1. Soak wakame in warm water for 5 minutes. Drain and squeeze out excess water. Chop into bite-sized pieces.
2. In a bowl, whisk together soy sauce, rice vinegar, mirin (if using), sugar, ginger, garlic, sesame oil, and red pepper flakes.
3. Add seaweed, cucumber, and sesame seeds to the dressing. Toss to combine. Serve immediately.

Nutrition Facts

Servings: 4

Amount per serving

Calories 139

	% Daily Value*
Total Fat 4.5g	6%
Saturated Fat 0.6g	3%
Cholesterol 0mg	0%
Sodium 504mg	22%
Total Carbohydrate 22.4g	8%
Dietary Fiber 0.7g	3%
Total Sugars 2.8g	
Protein 2.8g	
Vitamin D 0mcg	0%
Calcium 31mg	2%
Iron 1mg	4%
Potassium 35mg	1%

*The % Daily Value (DV) tells you how much a nutrient in a food serving contributes to a daily diet. 2,000 calorie a day is used for general nutrition advice.

Recipe analyzed by verywell

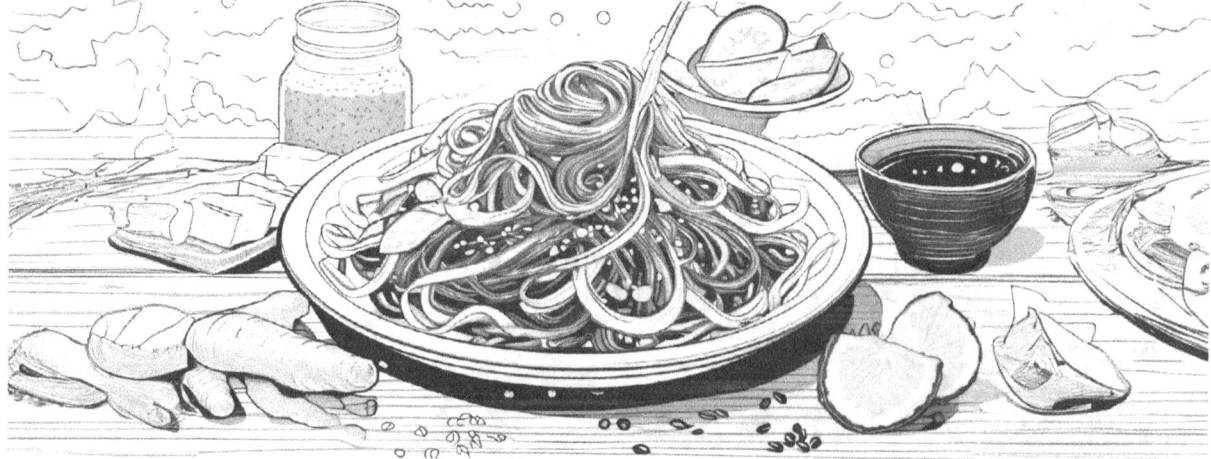

Simple Veggie Sautés

Simple Veggie Sautés offer a delightful and efficient way to get vegetables like spinach, zucchini, green beans, and more. Begin by heating a few tablespoons of avocado oil, then sauté the sliced onions and minced garlic until fragrant. Spinach wilts easily and only needs a sprinkle of salt and pepper. Green beans and zucchini, on the other hand, should be cooked to the desired doneness. Sauté the green beans quickly for a tender-crisp texture, and the zucchini should be sautéed quickly on each side to golden. This method brings out the natural flavors and nutrients in your veggies really quickly and healthily.

Ingredients

- Avocado Oil
- 1/2 of a Onion (sliced)
- 1/4 Cup Hemp Seeds
- Minced Garlic
- Salt and Pepper to taste
- Your Choice of Fresh Veggies: Spinach, Green Beans, Kale, Amaranth, Dandelion Greens, Collard Greens, Zucchini, Turnip, Purslane

Instructions

1. All you have to do is heat up a few tablespoons of neutral oil (avocado oil), add a 1/2 of a onion (sliced), some minced garlic and then add your vegetable(s) of choice. Spinach cooks the quickest, once it's wilted salt and pepper to taste.

2. Green beans I would follow the same steps. I personally prefer a snappier green bean so I don't cook them for long.

3. I also follow the same method for Zucchini and cook until they're brown on both sides.

Nutrition Facts

Serving size: Cups
Servings: 4

Amount per serving
Calories   **298**

% Daily Value*

Total Fat 8g	10%
Saturated Fat 1.8g	9%
Cholesterol 0mg	0%
Sodium 89mg	4%
Total Carbohydrate 54.3g	20%
Dietary Fiber 15.1g	54%
Total Sugars 3.5g	
Protein 11.8g	
Vitamin D 0mcg	0%
Calcium 325mg	25%
Iron 12mg	65%
Potassium 1146mg	24%

*The % Daily Value (DV) tells you how much a nutrient in a food serving contributes to a daily diet. 2,000 calorie a day is used for general nutrition advice.

Recipe analyzed by 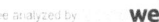 **well**

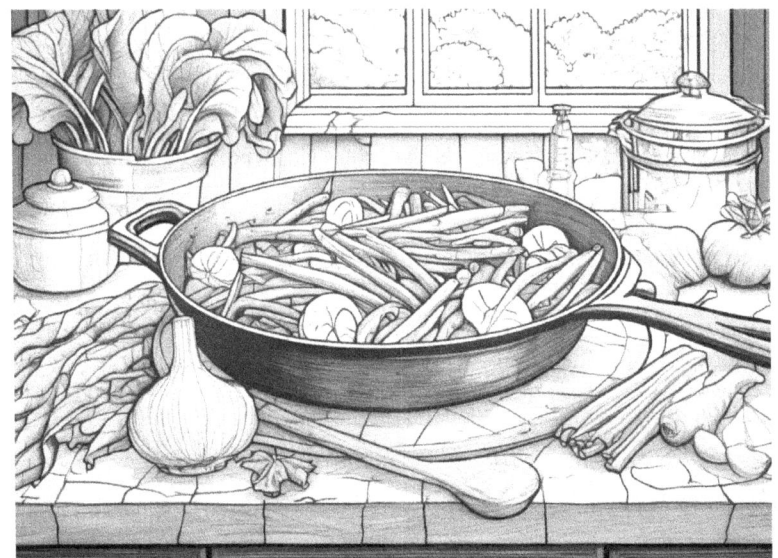

Ch 2: Soups + Sauces : Veggie Saute

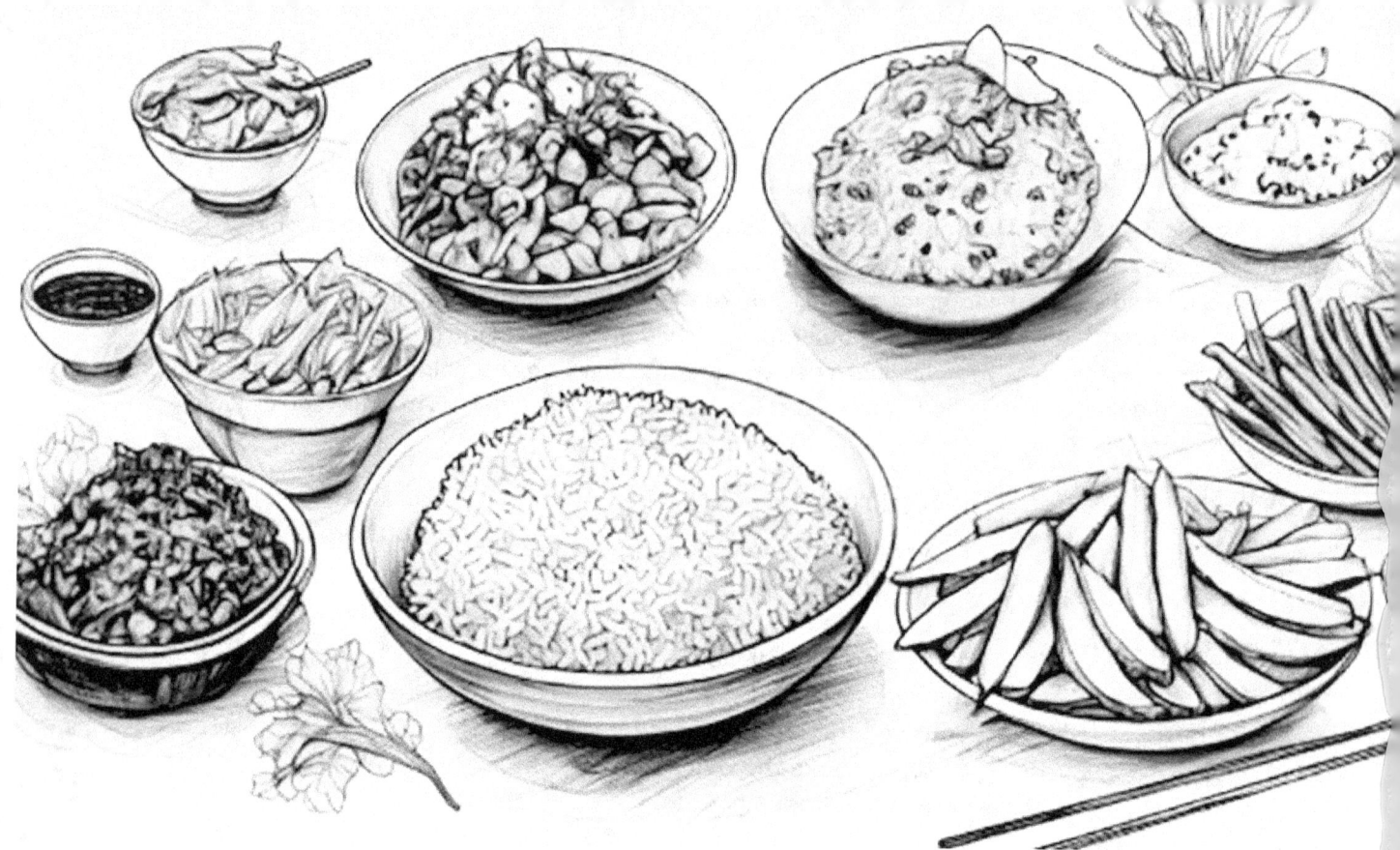

4.
INDIGENOUS RICES
AND
GRAINS

This section highlights a variety of rice and grain dishes, each crafted to bring out the unique taste and nutritional benefits of these essential ingredients. The Garlic Turmeric Rice blends the subtle floral notes of Jasmine rice with bold garlic and turmeric, creating a colorful and aromatic dish rich in healthy nutrients. Indigenous American Rice, or Arroz con Gandules, pays homage to Caribbean cuisine with a robust sofrito base, enriched by pitted olives, Sazón, gandules, and tomato sauce, resulting in a hearty, flavorful dish. Manchurian Fried Rice offers an elegant twist on traditional fried rice, infusing it with sweet onions, peas, carrots, and bean sprouts, all brought together with soy sauce and vegan oyster sauce for a savory umami experience. For a unique take on fries, Burro Fries or Fried Plantains provide a crunchy, delicious alternative using green Burro bananas or highly ripe plantains, each offering distinct textures and flavors. These recipes celebrate the diversity and richness of indigenous rices and grains, inviting you to explore and enjoy the depth of plant-based cuisine.

Garlic Turmeric Rice

Garlic Turmeric Rice is colorful, aromatic, and fuses subtle floral Jasmine rice flavors with bold garlic and turmeric. Begin by heating avocado oil in a saucepan. Add finely chopped shallots and garlic, and sauté until golden and fragrant. Mix in the Jasmine rice to coat with the oil and aromatics. Add turmeric and salt, incorporating well for even coloring. Next, add veggie or no-chicken broth and bring to a boil. Reduce the flame, cover, and cook until the rice is tender and the liquid is absorbed. Not only does it give the rice a nice golden color, but it also makes this dish rich in healthy nutrients from turmeric, making your meal tasty and nutritious at the same time.

Ingredients

- 2 - 4 cloves of garlic
- 1 - 3 shallots
- 1 cup Jasmine rice
- 2 cups veggie or no-chicken broth (I used no chicken this time)
- 1 tsp turmeric
- 1 tsp salt
- 2 tbsps oil (I used avocado oil)

Instructions

1. In a pan, heat the oil. Add the shallots and sauté. Add the garlic and the turmeric, and continue sautéing
2. Add the uncooked rice, toasting for 5 minutes (until all of the rice is coated with turmeric).
3. Add 1 3/4 cups of broth, salt and pepper to taste, then finish cook rice according to the instructions.

Nutrition Facts

Serving size: 1/2 Cup
Servings: 8

Amount per serving

Calories   89

% Daily Value*

Total Fat 5.9g	8%
Saturated Fat 1.2g	6%
Cholesterol 0mg	0%
Sodium 349mg	15%
Total Carbohydrate 8.8g	3%
Dietary Fiber 2.5g	9%
Total Sugars 0.4g	
Protein 1.2g	
Vitamin D 0mcg	0%
Calcium 12mg	1%
Iron 1mg	3%
Potassium 172mg	4%

*The % Daily Value (DV) tells you how much a nutrient in a food serving contributes to a daily diet. 2,000 calorie a day is used for general nutrition advice.

Recipe analyzed by **well**

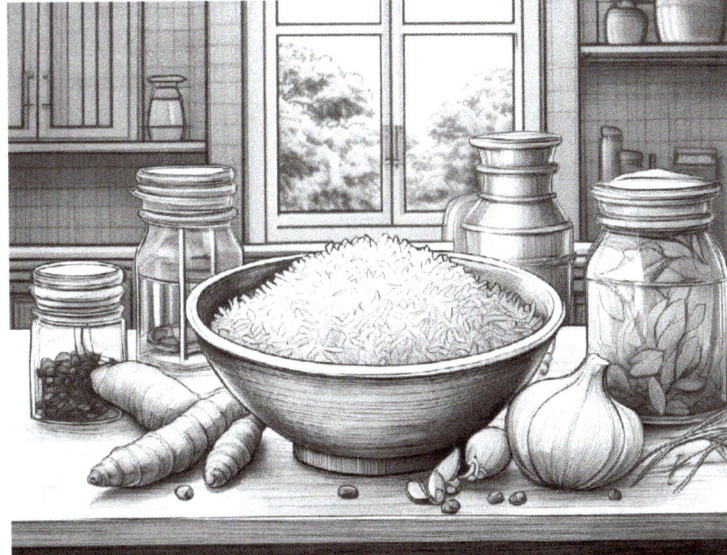

Ch 1: 5ntrees : Garlic Rice

Indigenous American Rice (Arroz con Gandules)

Indigenous American Rice, or Arroz con Gandules, is a classic dish rooted in the culinary traditions of the Americas, particularly celebrated in Caribbean cuisine. This recipe starts with the robust base of sofrito, a flavorful blend of herbs and vegetables that sets the foundational taste. To this, add pitted manzanilla olives and a packet of Sazón with culantro and achiote, enhancing the rice with vibrant color and deep flavors. Mix in gandules (pigeon peas), tomato sauce, and water, bringing the combination to a simmer before stirring in the rinsed white rice. Season with salt to taste. As the rice cooks, it absorbs the rich, aromatic flavors, resulting in a hearty, colorful dish that pays homage to its Indigenous American roots while delighting a diverse array of palates.

Nutrition Facts

Serving size: 1/2 Cup
Servings: 12

Amount per serving
Calories 810

	% Daily Value*
Total Fat 12.8g	16%
Saturated Fat 2.2g	11%
Cholesterol 0mg	0%
Sodium 5016mg	218%
Total Carbohydrate 134.7g	49%
Dietary Fiber 14.4g	51%
Total Sugars 3.6g	
Protein 32.8g	
Vitamin D 0mcg	0%
Calcium 162mg	12%
Iron 8mg	47%
Potassium 409mg	9%

*The % Daily Value (DV) tells you how much a nutrient in a food serving contributes to a daily diet. 2,000 calorie a day is used for general nutrition advice.

Recipe analyzed by verywell

Ingredients

- 1 can of gandules (drain liquid first)
- 12 Manzanilla Olives ***REMOVE PITS***
- 4 tbsp Sofrito
- 1 packet of Sazón (con Culantro y Achiote)
- 1 1/2 tbsp salt
- 8 ounce can of tomato sauce
- 4 cups of water
- 4 cups of rinsed white rice

Instruction

1. Warm pot (use a low flame). Add enough oil to cover the bottom of the pot (about 6 tbsp) and turn heat to high.

2. Add rice. Once it starts to boil, stir every couple of minutes so rice doesn't stick to the bottom of the pot.

3. After the rice has soaked up all the ingredients, lower flame, cover the pot and let it cook for 55 minutes.

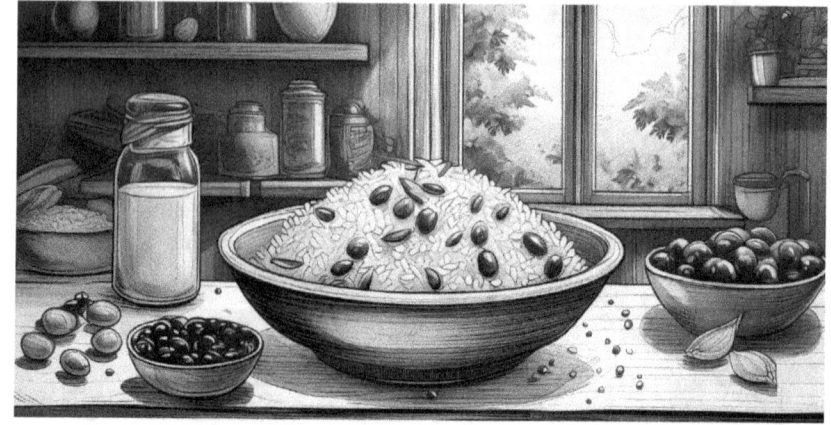

Ch 5: Entrees : Arroz con Gandules

Fried Rice (Manchurian)

Manchurian Fried Rice is an elegant twist on the usual fried rice, created with a cross-infusion of flavors that really zing the taste buds. Heat toasted sesame oil in a large pan or wok. Add chopped sweet onion and cook until translucent. Toss in frozen peas and carrots with bean sprouts and cook until the peas and carrots are just tender. Add the day-old rice that's been separated. Pour in soy sauce or liquid aminos, vegan oyster sauce, and a sprinkle of white pepper for just a hint of heat. Stir well, coating the rice and heating it through so the savory, umami flavors meld together. This Manchurian Fried Rice is one creative dish with vegan ingredients that's perfectly hearty.

Ingredients

- 3 Cup Day Old Rice
- 1 Cup Frozen Peas and Carrots
- 1/2 Cup Bean Sprouts
- 1/2 Large Sweet Onion
- 1 Tsp Toasted Sesame Oil
- 3 Tbsp Soy Sauce / Liquid Aminos
- 1 1/2 Tbsp Vegan Oyster Sauce
- 1/2 Tsp White Pepper

Instructions

1. Start by heating neutral oil (Avocado oil) in a wok (pans can work too).
2. Add onion and sauté until almost translucent, followed by bean sprouts.
3. Add rice being sure allow frying.
4. Next, add sesame oil, soy sauce, oyster sauce and white pepper. Stir well to combine.
5. Lastly add frozen peas & carrots and continue mixing until they are tender.

Nutrition Facts

Serving size: 1/2 Cup
Servings: 8

Amount per serving
Calories 95

	% Daily Value*
Total Fat 1.9g	2%
Saturated Fat 0.1g	0%
Cholesterol 0mg	0%
Sodium 2582mg	112%
Total Carbohydrate 18.7g	7%
Dietary Fiber 0.7g	2%
Total Sugars 1.3g	
Protein 6.6g	
Vitamin D 0mcg	0%
Calcium 4mg	0%
Iron 4mg	20%
Potassium 39mg	1%

*The % Daily Value (DV) tells you how much a nutrient in a food serving contributes to a daily diet. 2,000 calorie a day is used for general nutrition advice.

Recipe analyzed by **well**

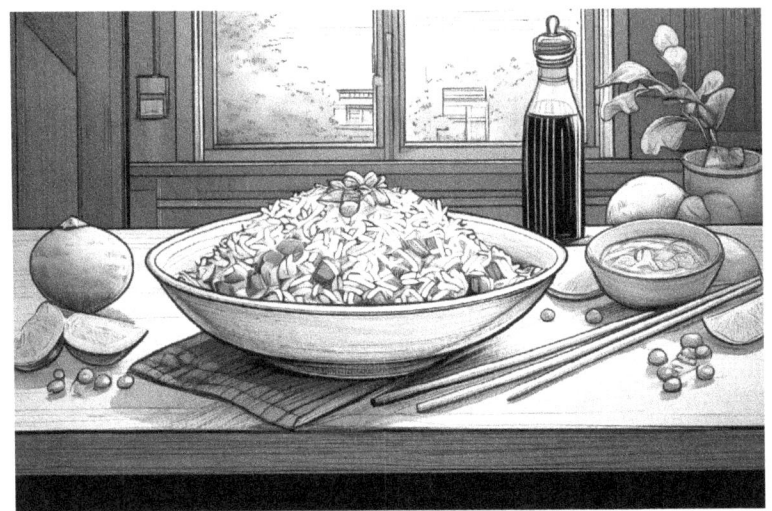

Ch 1: 5ntrees : Arroz con Gandules

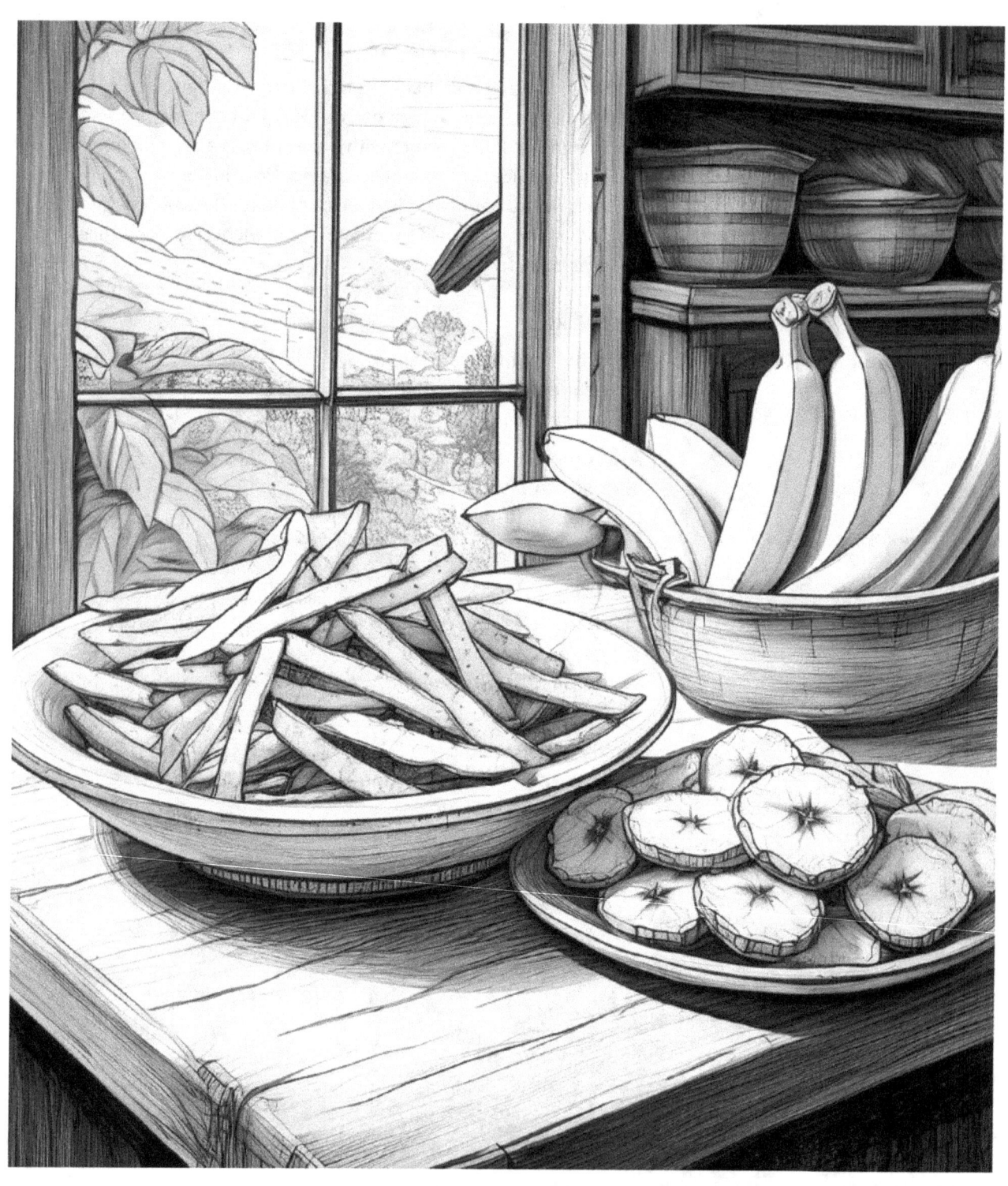

Ch 5: Entrees : Burro Fries/ Plantain

Burro Fries / Fried Plantain

Burro Fries: are a tasty break from ordinary fries. These fries are made from green Burro bananas. This simple yet inventive recipe brings a firm texture to a dish that's crunchy and delicious at the same time. It's made by cutting the bananas into fry-like shapes, then soaking them in cold water to remove any excess starch that would have made them softer instead of crunchy when fried. On the other hand, for fried plantains, you want to select highly ripe ones, nearly black; that ripeness ensures they're sweet and tender, allowing you to develop a caramelized exterior when frying. Whether you choose Burro bananas or ripe plantains, this recipe dares you to find an unexpectedly delicious way to enjoy these versatile fruits, making you think twice before ever ordering them in a restaurant.

Ingredients

- Green (Unripe) Burro Bananas or VERY Ripe Plantains

Instructions

1. Peel, cut diagonally, soak in cold water and fry until golden.
2. Drain, then lightly sprinkle with salt.

Nutrition Facts (Burro Banana)

Serving size: 1 Banana
Servings: 4

Amount per serving
Calories 131

	% Daily Value*
Total Fat 4.9g	6%
Saturated Fat 1g	5%
Cholesterol 0mg	0%
Sodium 2mg	0%
Total Carbohydrate 22.2g	8%
Dietary Fiber 2.7g	10%
Total Sugars 13.1g	
Protein 1.5g	
Vitamin D 0mcg	0%
Calcium 3mg	0%
Iron 0mg	1%
Potassium 121mg	3%

*The % Daily Value (DV) tells you how much a nutrient in a food serving contributes to a daily diet. 2,000 calorie a day is used for general nutrition advice.

Recipe analyzed by well

Nutrition Facts (Plantain)

Serving size: 1 Plantain
Servings: 4

Amount per serving
Calories 135

	% Daily Value*
Total Fat 1.6g	2%
Saturated Fat 0.4g	2%
Cholesterol 0mg	0%
Sodium 4mg	0%
Total Carbohydrate 32.4g	12%
Dietary Fiber 2.7g	10%
Total Sugars 15g	
Protein 1.4g	
Vitamin D 0mcg	0%
Calcium 4mg	0%
Iron 1mg	4%
Potassium 529mg	11%

*The % Daily Value (DV) tells you how much a nutrient in a food serving contributes to a daily diet. 2,000 calorie a day is used for general nutrition advice.

Recipe analyzed by well

Notes

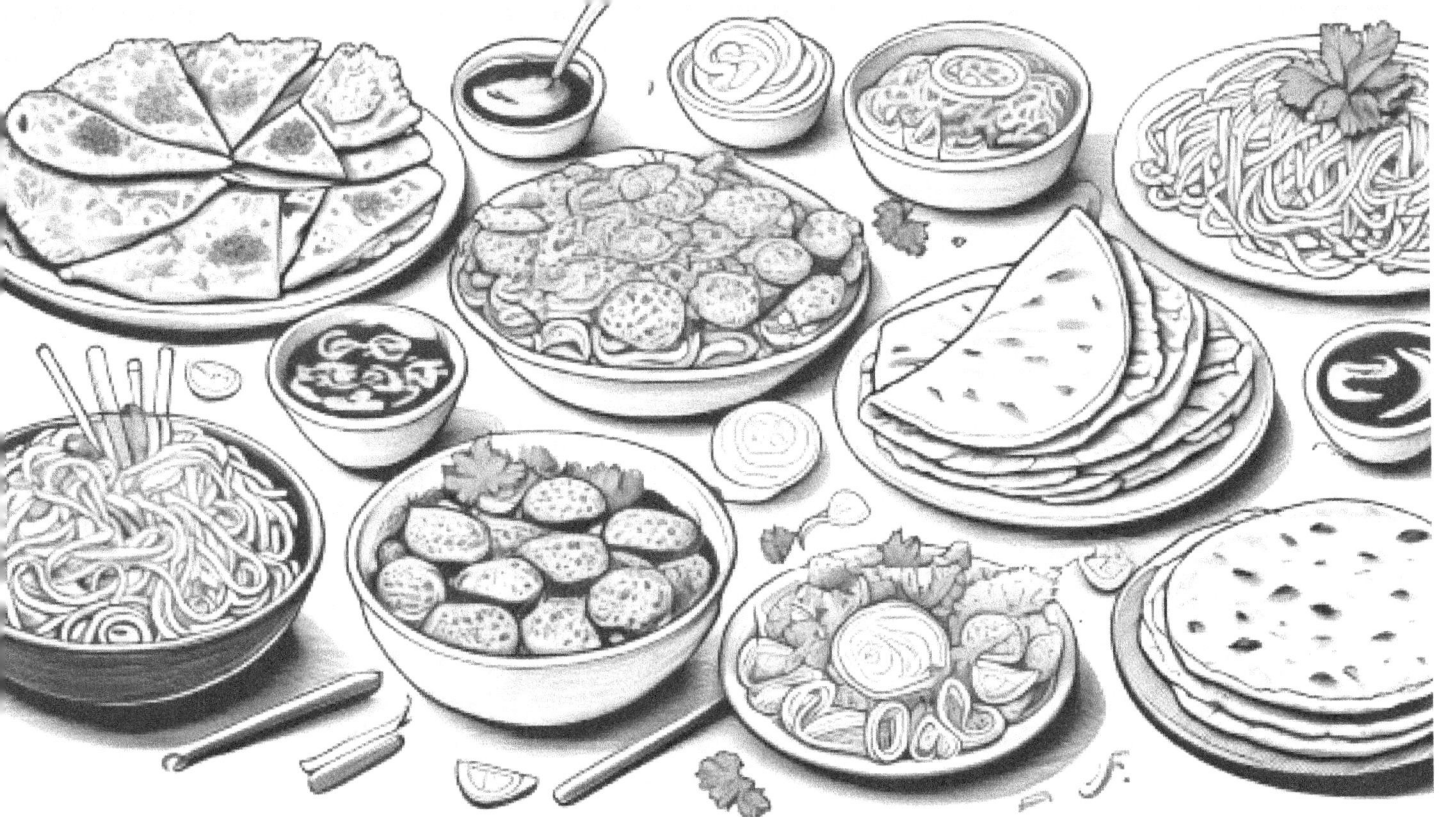

5.

ENTREES
PICK YOUR PROTEIN

This section offers a diverse range of recipes, each designed to bring out the best in vegan cooking. For breakfast enthusiasts, light and fluffy pancakes and waffles set the stage for a delightful morning start. Middle Eastern cuisine lovers will appreciate the crispy, savory falafel, transforming simple chickpeas into a delightful dish. For those craving bold, smoky flavors, recipes like BBQ Jackfruit and Jerk Veggies provide delicious alternatives, celebrating the rich, hearty essence of barbecue and Caribbean spice. The versatile jackfruit also shines in salads and tacos, offering creamy, tangy twists and vibrant, satisfying meals. Asian-inspired dishes such as Asiatic Mixed Veggies and Noodles in Brown Sauce bring together colorful vegetables and hearty noodles for a fusion of flavors. Classic comfort foods are reimagined with vegan pasta options like red sauce, creamy Alfredo, and pesto, highlighting traditional tastes with a modern twist. Innovative takes on seafood, such as Lion's Mane Mushroom Crab Cake, showcase the possibilities of plant-based ingredients. Lastly, hearty wraps, sandwiches, and the iconic Chopped Cheese offer satisfying, innovative meals that honor culinary traditions while embracing healthy, modern eating. Dive into these recipes and explore the delicious possibilities of vegan cuisine.

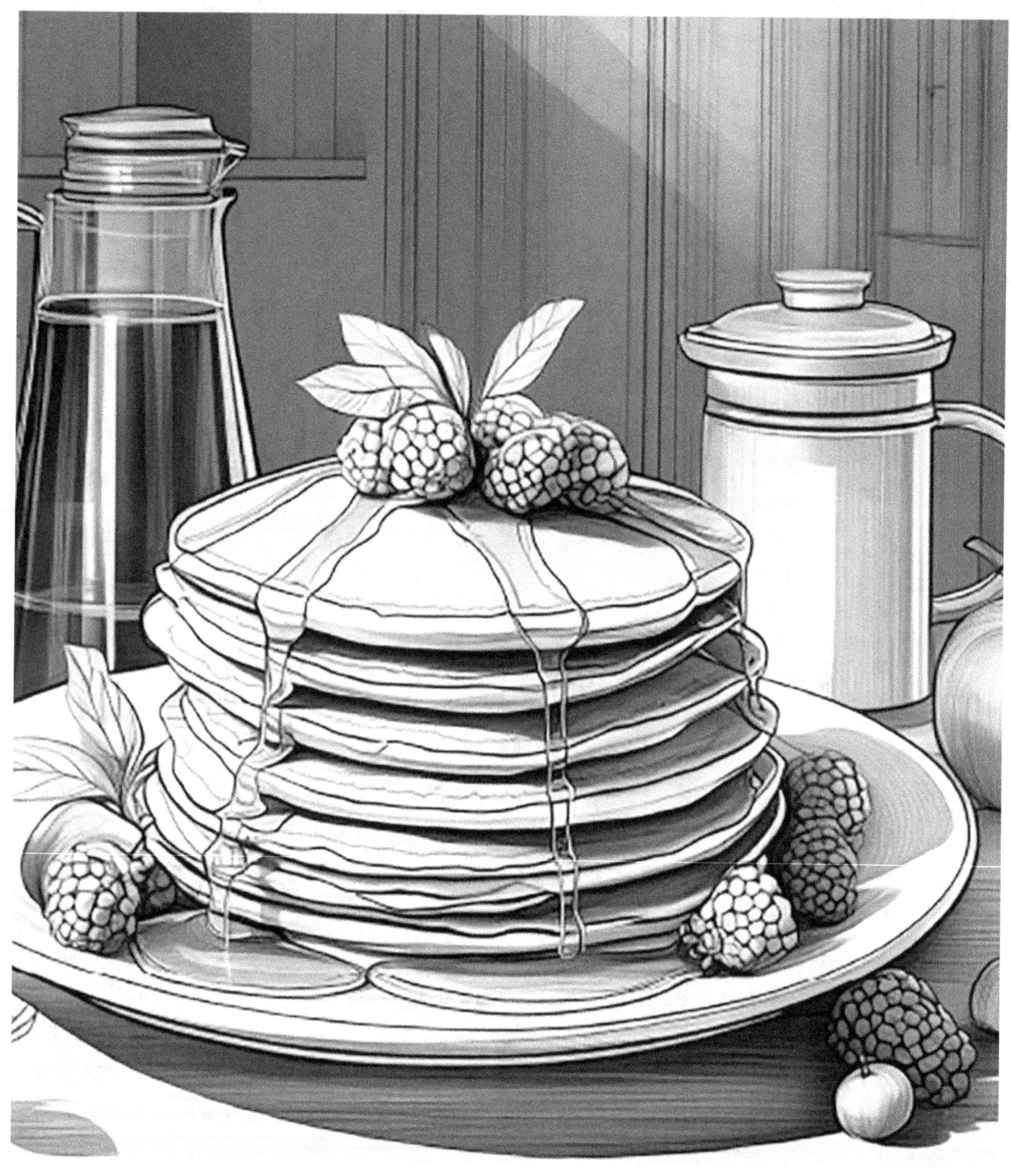

Ch 5: Entrees : Pancakes

Pancakes / Waffles

Pancakes and waffles: breakfast favorites, made easily, vegan-style, without sacrificing any taste or texture. hisk together some all-purWpose flour, baking powder, a pinch of salt, and some granulated sugar. Gradually whisk in soy milk, water, and maybe a tiny bit of canola oil if you prefer that - I usually skip the oil in mine and think they're just as light and fluffy. For pancakes, pour the batter on a hot griddle or frying pan and cook until bubbles form and the edges look set before flipping. For waffles, cook the batter in a heated waffle iron until golden and crispy. Serve with all your favorite toppings for a light, fluffy, tasty breakfast treat.

Ingredients

- 1 1/2 Cups All Purpose Flour *See Notes For Options
- 1 Tablespoon Baking Powder
- 1/2 Teaspoon Salt
- 2 Tablespoons Granulated Sugar
- 1 Cup Soy Milk *Or Use Almond, Oat Or Coconut Milk 1/2 Cup
- Water
- 2 Tablespoons Canola Oil *May Omit For Oil Free

Instructions

1. Start by mixing wet ingredients in a medium bowl and set to the side.
2. In a large bowl, sift flour and baking powder. Add sugar and salt then gently whisk to evenly combine.
3. Pour the wet mixture into the large bowl and mix gently being sure not to over mix. ***This is one pancake recipe that you want to see clumps in.***
4. Heat a large griddle or pan over medium-high heat. Grease the pan with vegan butter or coconut oil, and drop about 1/3 cup of the batter onto it.
5. Cook until bubbles form, then flip and cook until golden brown on the other side, about 1-2 minutes.
6. Repeat with all the remaining batter. Serve with vegan butter, pure maple syrup and fresh fruit.

Nutrition Facts

Serving size: 4 Pancakes
Servings: 16

Amount per serving

Calories 110

% Daily Value*

Total Fat 2.3g	3%
Saturated Fat 0.3g	2%
Cholesterol 0mg	0%
Sodium 1266mg	55%
Total Carbohydrate 22g	8%
Dietary Fiber 1.4g	5%
Total Sugars 13.4g	
Protein 1.7g	
Vitamin D 0mcg	0%
Calcium 35mg	3%
Iron 1mg	3%
Potassium 56mg	1%

*The % Daily Value (DV) tells you how much a nutrient in a food serving contributes to a daily diet. 2,000 calorie a day is used for general nutrition advice.

Recipe analyzed by **well**

Falafel

Falafel, a beloved Middle Eastern dish, is a delightful way to enjoy plant-based cuisine. Begin by soaking dried garbanzo beans overnight until tender. Drain and blend them with diced yellow onion, minced garlic, and a chopped Italian herb blend. Add cumin, ground coriander, cayenne pepper, and baking soda to enhance flavor and texture. Incorporate the juice of half a key lime and chickpea flour, mixing until well combined. Season with salt and pepper to taste. Shape the mixture into balls or patties and fry until golden brown. Enjoy these crispy, flavorful falafel in a wrap, salad, or on their own with a dipping sauce. Interesting Fact: Falafel is thought to have originated in Egypt, where it was made with fava beans. It has since become a staple street food across the Middle East, with each region adding its own unique twist to this ancient recipe.

Ingredients

- 1 Cup Dried Garbanzo Beans (Chickpeas)
- 1/2 Yellow Onion (Diced)
- 4 Cloves Minced Garlic
- 1/2 Cup Chopped Italian Herb Blend
- 1 Tsp Cumin
- 1/2 Tsp Ground Coriander
- 1/8 Tsp Cayenne Pepper
- 1/4 Tsp Baking Soda
- 1/2 Key Lime (Juiced)
- 1 Tbsp Chickpea Flour
- Salt And Pepper To Taste

Instructions

1. If you using dried chickpeas, start by soaking chickpeas overnight in advance
2. Strain soaked or canned chickpeas.
3. Add all ingredients to food processor. Pulse about 50 times (yes, I've counted) to maintain a small / ground consistency. Mixture should not too smooth.
4. Refrigerate for an hour. Form chilled mixture into balls or patties. Wetting hands with water will make forming the falafel a bit easier.
5. Fry at 350°F for about 5 minutes or until browned and crispy.
6. Serve with tahini, pita, and fresh veggies.

Nutrition Facts

Serving size: 3 - 4 Pieces
Servings: 12

Amount per serving

Calories   101

	% Daily Value*
Total Fat 1.7g	2%
Saturated Fat 0.2g	1%
Cholesterol 0mg	0%
Sodium 40mg	2%
Total Carbohydrate 16.6g	6%
Dietary Fiber 4.1g	15%
Total Sugars 2.9g	
Protein 5.4g	
Vitamin D 0mcg	0%
Calcium 32mg	2%
Iron 2mg	9%
Potassium 259mg	6%

*The % Daily Value (DV) tells you how much a nutrient in a food serving contributes to a daily diet. 2,000 calorie a day is used for general nutrition advice.

Recipe analyzed by verywell

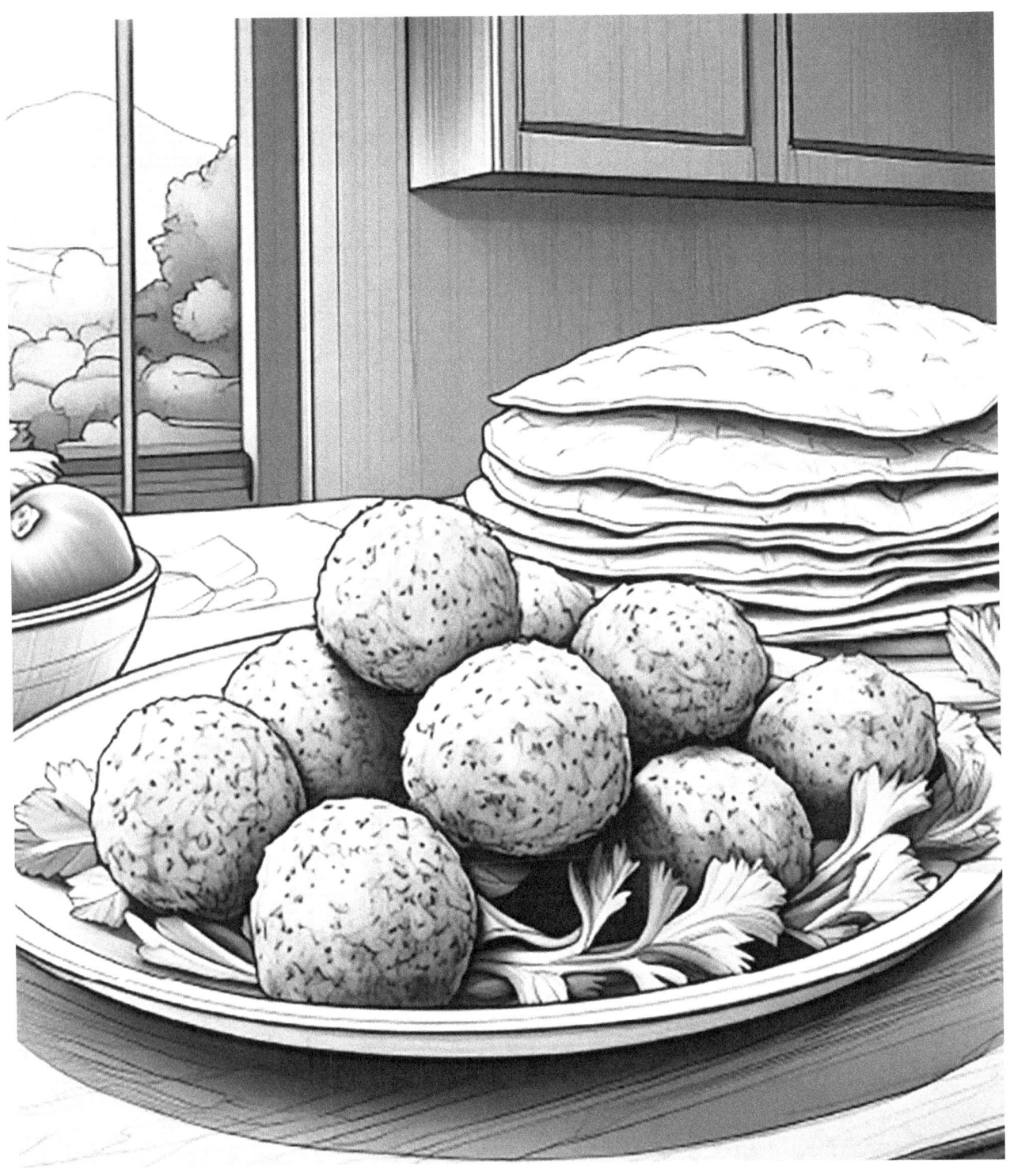

Ch 5: Entrees : Falafel

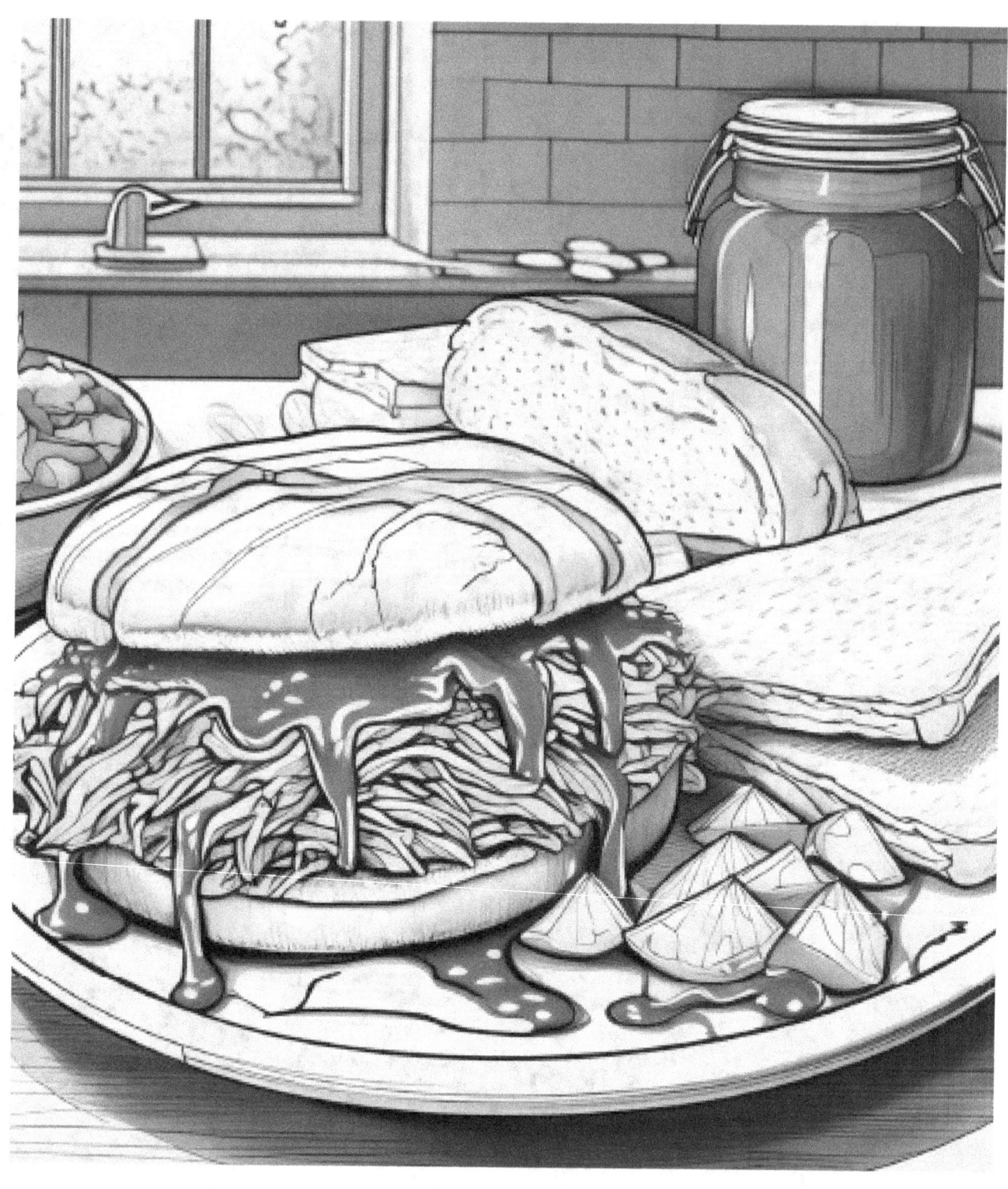

Ch 5: Entrees : BBQ Jackfruit

BBQ Jackfruit

BBQ jackfruit flips plant-based cooking on its head with the bold, smoky flavors of a barbecue dish, suitable for even vegans. As such, it has been taken up with a relish by the Moorish–American community as it explores and reimagines traditional recipes, holding them up to different lenses of a healthier, sometimes vegan diet without losing strong deep flavors. Heavily seasoned with sazón and adobo, garlic and onion powders, and a very generous slather of BBQ sauce, the final result is that kind of sandwich which reveals just how sweet and intensely savory the flavors can get—really tough competition for any pulled pork. It celebrates the spirit of innovation and creativity in the Moorish American tradition. So dig into this BBQ Jackfruit and enjoy a history lesson dripping with flavor.

Ingredients

- 1 Can Organic Young Jackfruit
- 1/2 Packet Of Sazon
- 2 Tbsp Adobo
- 2 Tbsp Garlic Powder
- 2 Tbsp Onion Powder
- 1/2 - 3/4 Cup Of Bbq Sauce

Instructions

1. Start by putting jackfruit in saucepan and cover with water. Boil until jackfruit starts to separate then simmer for 5-7 minutes.
2. Drain jackfruit and return to pan. Add water to almost cover and add sazon.
3. Bring to boil then simmer for 5 minutes or until the liquid evaporates, stirring regularly and pressing with a fork to shred the pieces.
4. Add adobo, garlic powder, onion powder, and BBQ sauce.
5. Simmer 5 more minutes, then serve on pita or your favorite roll.
6. Add the coleslaw from the salad section of this book for a sandwich that you will absolutely want to keep in your rotation.

Nutrition Facts

Serving size: 1/4 Cup
Servings: 8

Amount per serving

Calories — 183

	% Daily Value*
Total Fat 0.5g	1%
Saturated Fat 0.1g	0%
Cholesterol 0mg	0%
Sodium 717mg	31%
Total Carbohydrate 41.3g	15%
Dietary Fiber 4.6g	16%
Total Sugars 16.6g	
Protein 6.8g	
Vitamin D 0mcg	0%
Calcium 112mg	9%
Iron 2mg	10%
Potassium 524mg	11%

*The % Daily Value (DV) tells you how much a nutrient in a food serving contributes to a daily diet. 2,000 calorie a day is used for general nutrition advice.

Recipe analyzed by **well**

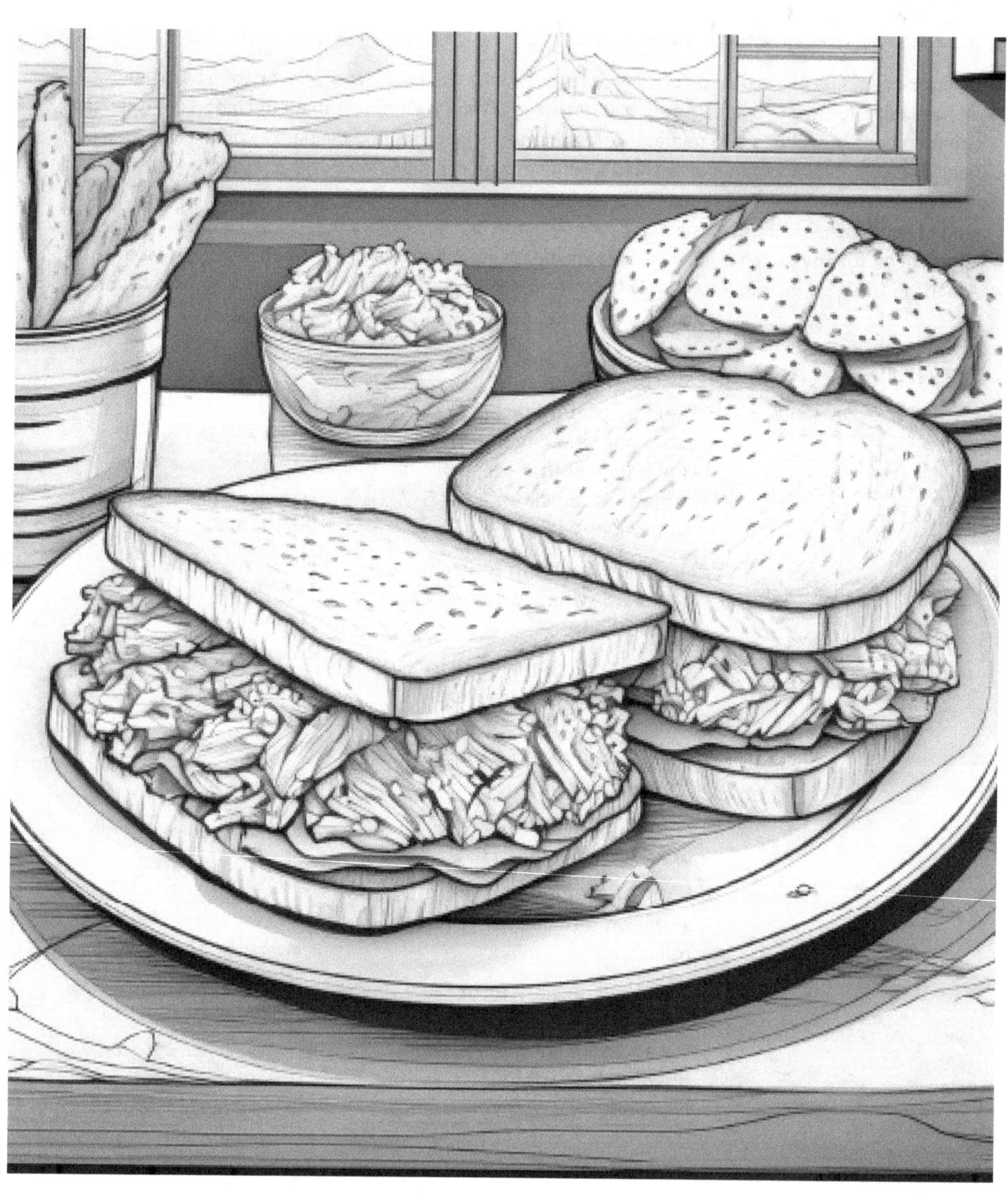

Ch 5: Entrées : Jackfruit Tuna/Chicken

Jackfruit Tuna/Chicken

Jackfruit Tuna/Chicken is a flexible, delicious, plant-based alternative that evokes classic tuna or chicken salad, only better. This versatile ingredient mimics meat and shines in vegan cooking, especially in Moorish American cuisine. In this recipe, tender shredded young jackfruit combines with a Not-Chick'n bouillon cube for savory depth. Chopped onion, sweet relish, vegan mayo, and spicy brown mustard create a creamy, tangy salad. Salt and pepper to taste, and serve on bread or in a wrap—it also dresses salad nicely. This plant-based recipe adds to the growing trend of converting classic dishes into healthier, plant-based forms. Jackfruit salad offers a bite of history and creativity.

Ingredients

- 1 Can Organic Young Jackfruit
- 1 Cube Not-Chick'n Bouillon Cubes
- 1/3 Cup Chopped Onion
- 1/3 Cup Sweet Relish
- 1/3 Cup Vegan Mayo
- 1/4 Cup Spicy Brown Mustard
- Salt And Pepper (To Taste)

Ingredients:

1. Start by putting jackfruit in saucepan and cover with water. Boil until jackfruit starts to separate, then simmer another 5-7 minutes.

2. Drain jackfruit and return to pan. Add water to cover and 1 bouillon cube. Bring to boil then simmer for 5 minutes, stirring regularly.

3. Drain and put jackfruit into bowl. Add mayonnaise, mustard, relish, onions, salt and pepper and mash while "stirring well to break up bigger chunks.

4. Serve with your favorite crackers, pita or as a sandwich on your favorite bread.

Nutrition Facts

Serving size: 1/4 Cup
Servings: 8

Amount per serving

Calories 48

	% Daily Value*
Total Fat 3.2g	4%
Saturated Fat 0.4g	2%
Cholesterol 0mg	0%
Sodium 251mg	11%
Total Carbohydrate 4.7g	2%
Dietary Fiber 0.8g	3%
Total Sugars 3.2g	
Protein 0.2g	
Vitamin D 0mcg	0%
Calcium 1mg	0%
Iron 1mg	3%
Potassium 10mg	0%

*The % Daily Value (DV) tells you how much a nutrient in a food serving contributes to a daily diet. 2,000 calorie a day is used for general nutrition advice.

Recipe analyzed by **well**

Jackfruit Veggie Tacos / Burritos

Jackfruit Veggie Tacos/Burritos are a vibrant, plant-based twist on classic Mexican cuisine, celebrating the rich flavors and textures of fresh vegetables and tender jackfruit. This recipe combines shredded organic young jackfruit with a colorful mix of green, red, yellow, and orange peppers, sweet onion, and zucchini, with optional mushrooms for added depth. Seasoned with a packet of Sazon, Adobo, garlic and onion powders, cumin, and a chili pepper in adobo sauce, these tacos or burritos are packed with bold, smoky flavors. Perfect for a healthy, satisfying meal, they showcase the innovative use of jackfruit in creating delicious, meat-free alternatives that honor traditional culinary roots while embracing modern, plant-based diets.

Ingredients

- 1 Can Organic Young Jackfruit
- 1 Green Pepper
- 1 Red Pepper
- 1 Yellow Pepper
- 1 Orange Pepper
- 1 Sweet Onion
- 1 Zucchini
- Mushrooms *Optional*
- 1 Packet Of Sazon
- 1 Tbsp Adobo
- 1 Tbsp Garlic Powder
- 1 Tbsp Onion Powder
- 2 Tbsp Cumin
- 1 Chili Pepper In Adobo Sauce
- 1 Tbsp Chili Pepper Adobo Sauce

Ingredients

1. Start by putting jackfruit in saucepan and cover with water. Boil until jackfruit starts to separate, then simmer another 5-7 minutes.
2. Drain jackfruit then return to pan. Add water to almost cover and add sazon. Bring to boil then simmer for 5 minutes or until the liquid reduces, stirring regularly and pressing with spatula to shred the pieces.
3. While the jackfruit is cooking, you may want to cut your peppers into strips and slice your onions, zucchini, and mushrooms if you are using them. Sauté veggies.
4. Transfer jackfruit and any left over liquid to pan with veggies. Add seasoning (adobo, garlic powder, onion powder and cumin) and minced chili pepper with adobo sauce.
5. Stir to combine and let simmer 2-3 minutes. Remove from heat and serve.

Nutrition Facts

Serving size: 1/2 Cup
Servings: 12

Amount per serving
Calories 31

	% Daily Value*
Total Fat 0.5g	1%
Saturated Fat 0g	0%
Cholesterol 2mg	1%
Sodium 578mg	25%
Total Carbohydrate 6.4g	2%
Dietary Fiber 2.6g	9%
Total Sugars 2.5g	
Protein 1.4g	
Vitamin D 0mcg	0%
Calcium 15mg	1%
Iron 2mg	9%
Potassium 156mg	3%

*The % Daily Value (DV) tells you how much a nutrient in a food serving contributes to a daily diet. 2,000 calorie a day is used for general nutrition advice.

Recipe analyzed by **verywell**

Ch 5: Entrees : Jackfruit Tuna/Chicken

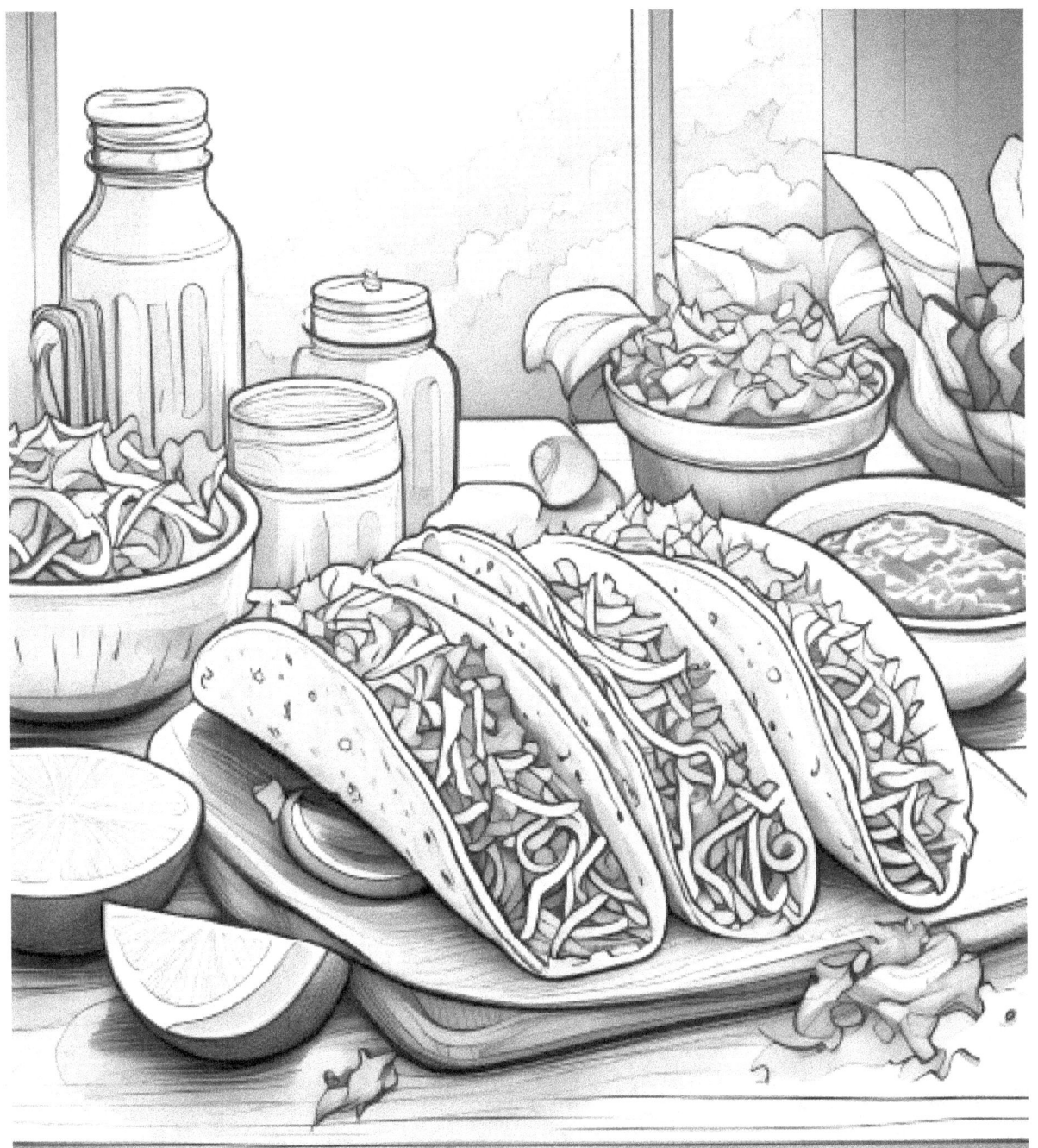

Garnish with lime and fresh cilantro. Serve as tacos with salsa and/or guacamole, lettuce, tomatoes, diced onions, vegan sour cream, arroz con gandules, and plantains.

To serve as burritos, fill burrito wrap with indigenous grain of your choice (arroz con gandules), jackfruit, veggies and wrap. Grill on both
sides. Serve with your favorite chips, fresh salsa and guacamole.
*Side note - Oyster or Trumpet mushrooms may be great replacements for jackfruit

Ch 5: Entrees : Jackfruit Tacos

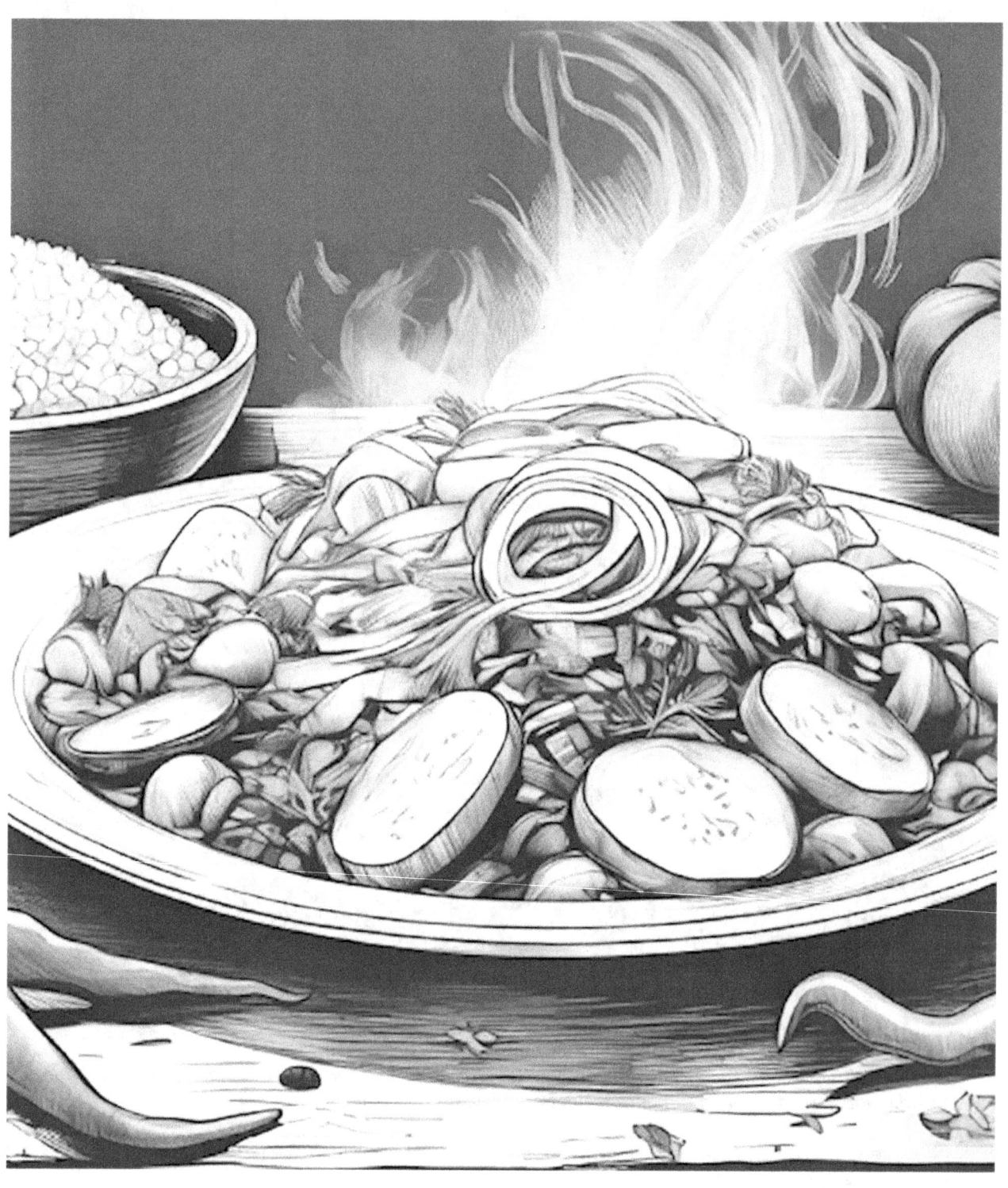

Jerk Veggies
Jackfruit / Mushrooms

Jerk Veggies with Jackfruit or Mushrooms brings the bold, spicy flavors of Caribbean cuisine to a plant-based dish. This recipe features organic young jackfruit or mushrooms combined with a vibrant mix of green, red, yellow, and orange peppers, sweet onion, and zucchini. Seasoned with Adobo and coated in rich, aromatic jerk sauce, these veggies are transformed into a deliciously spiced meal. Perfect for tacos, wraps, or served over rice, this dish celebrates the fusion of traditional Caribbean flavors with the innovative use of plant-based ingredients, offering a healthy and flavorful alternative that's sure to delight and satisfy.

Ingredients

- 1 Can Organic Young Jackfruit
- 1 Green Pepper
- 1 Red Pepper
- 1 Yellow Pepper
- 1 Orange Pepper
- 1 Sweet Onion
- 1 Zucchini
- 1 Tbsp Adobo
- 1/2 Cup Jerk Sauce
- Mushrooms *Optional* (Baby Bella, Oyster, King Oyster or Lion's Mane are all great options)

Instructions

1. Start by cubing your peppers and onions and slicing your zucchini (and mushrooms if you are using them). Add to large mixing bowl.
2. Lightly oil and add jerk sauce to marinate.
3. While veggies are marinating strain jackfruit and add to saucepan and cover with water. Boil until jackfruit starts to separate.
4. Simmer another 5-7 minutes. Drain jackfruit and return to pan.
5. Add water to almost cover and add adobo. Bring to boil then simmer for 5 minutes or until the liquid reduces, stirring regularly. This jackfruit we want to keep chunkier so no need to press and shred.
6. Add marinated veggies & jackfruit to a hot pan and sauté covered.
7. Serve hot with your choice of indigenous grains (fonio or quinoa) and enjoy.

Nutrition Facts

Serving size: 1 cup
Servings: 4

Amount per serving

Calories 55

	% Daily Value*
Total Fat 0.7g	1%
Saturated Fat 0g	0%
Cholesterol 0mg	0%
Sodium 8087mg	352%
Total Carbohydrate 11g	4%
Dietary Fiber 4.3g	15%
Total Sugars 3.8g	
Protein 2.6g	
Vitamin D 90mcg	450%
Calcium 16mg	1%
Iron 1mg	8%
Potassium 322mg	7%

*The % Daily Value (DV) tells you how much a nutrient in a food serving contributes to a daily diet. 2,000 calorie a day is used for general nutrition advice.

Recipe analyzed by **well**

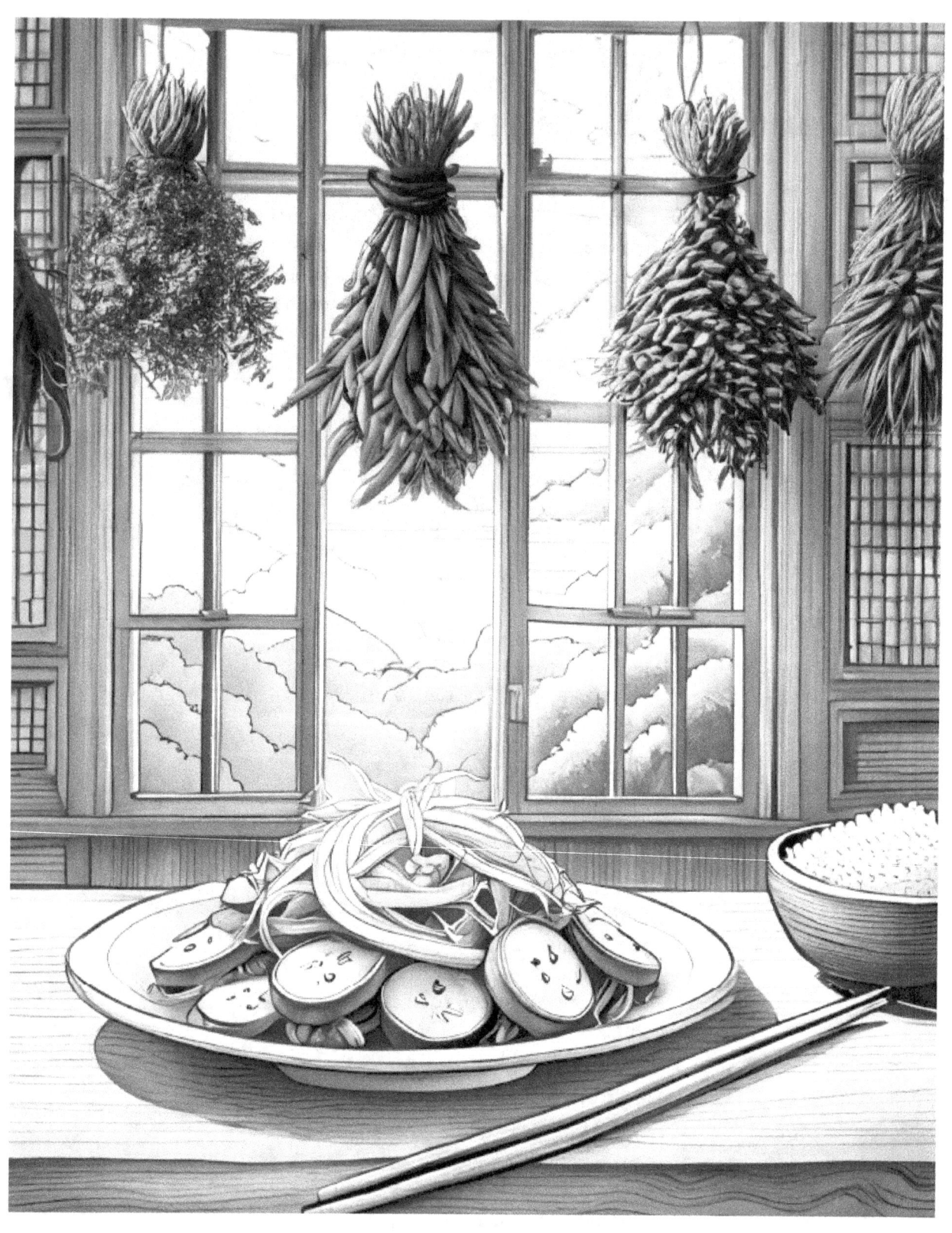

Ch 5: Entrees : Asiatic Mixed Veggies

Asiatic Mixed Veggies
Brown Sauce (Manchurian)

Asiatic Mixed Veggies is a colorful and tasty dish that boasts the hues of fresh, vibrant vegetables. This is an evident example of culinary art that exists amidst the Moorish Americans, and its inspiration and intuition compose the taste coming from different peppers, sweet onion, zucchini, and mushrooms, if desired. All of these have their own texture and taste, combined in a symphony that is both visually pleasant and tastes divine. Stir-fried just right, this dish portrays the grand tradition of combining mixed vegetables with a vast array of ingredients. Enjoy this with Manchurian Sauce as a main course or delightful side that celebrates a fusion of cultures and a commitment to healthy, flavorful eating.

Ingredients

- 1 Green Pepper
- 1 Red Pepper
- 1 Yellow Pepper
- 1 Orange Pepper
- 1 Sweet Onion
- 1 Zucchini
- Mushrooms *Optional*

Instructions

1. Strip or cube vegetables.
2. Heat a pan or wok then add a couple tablespoons of avocado (neutral) oil.
3. Add veggies and sauté until onion is almost translucent (I like a snap to my veggies).
4. Remove veggies from pan or wok to a heat-proof bowl. Add the brown sauce from the sauces section of this book and allow sauce to heat up slightly bubbling, then add vegetables back to the pan or wok and evenly coat.
5. Serve with any side from the sides section of this book or indigenous rices / grains for a multi course meal.

Nutrition Facts

Serving size: 1 cup
Servings: 4

Amount per serving

Calories   55

	% Daily Value*
Total Fat 0.7g	1%
Saturated Fat 0g	0%
Cholesterol 0mg	0%
Sodium 8087mg	352%
Total Carbohydrate 11g	4%
Dietary Fiber 4.3g	15%
Total Sugars 3.8g	
Protein 2.6g	
Vitamin D 90mcg	450%
Calcium 16mg	1%
Iron 1mg	8%
Potassium 322mg	7%

*The % Daily Value (DV) tells you how much a nutrient in a food serving contributes to a daily diet. 2,000 calorie a day is used for general nutrition advice.

Recipe analyzed by **well**

Noodles in Brown Sauce (Manchurian)

This recipe is a great example of how the knowledge of sauces, coupled with an openness to explore ingredients found in local markets and a willingness to experiment in the kitchen, can lead to a fun and fulfilling culinary experience. Noodles in Brown Sauce is a savory and satisfying medley of fresh vegetables and hearty udon noodles, highlighting the fusion of flavors and the embrace of plant-based ingredients. The dish showcases the chef's creativity in combining various elements to create a harmonious and delectable meal. By honoring traditional Asian influences and incorporating them into a modern context, this recipe offers a delicious and wholesome dish that bridges cultures and flavors, demonstrating the power of food to unite people and celebrate diversity. This Noodles in Brown Sauce recipe is a testament to the joy and satisfaction that can be found in exploring new ingredients, techniques, and flavor combinations in the kitchen.

Ingredients

- 1 Tbsp Ginger Paste
- 1 Tbsp Roasted Minced Garlic
- 1 Tbsp Chinese 5 Spice
- 1 Green Pepper
- 1 Red Pepper
- 1 Yellow Pepper
- 1 Orange Pepper
- 1 Sweet Onion
- 1 Zucchini
- 1 Cup Mung Bean Sprouts
- Mushrooms *Optional*
- 1 Pack Udon Noodles
- 1/2 Cup Brown Sauce

Instructions

1. Sauté your veggies using a neutral oil. Lightly season with Chinese 5 spice, ginger, garlic and onion then set aside.
2. Cook your favorite noodles (ramen, soba, lo mein, udon, etc) using the directions on the package.
3. After noodles are cooked, (usually rinsed in cold water) and set to the side, in a wok (or pan) heat up oil and pour in sauce.
4. Once the sauce starts to bubble and thicken, add cooked veggies and noodles. Stir until everything is coated and serve.
5. Garnish with green onions and sesame seeds.
6. Serve with seaweed salad found in the Sides section of this cookbook.

Nutrition Facts

Serving size: 1 cup
Servings: 4

Amount per serving
Calories — **250**

	% Daily Value*
Total Fat 3.9g	5%
Saturated Fat 0.6g	3%
Cholesterol 0mg	0%
Sodium 315mg	14%
Total Carbohydrate 50.6g	18%
Dietary Fiber 8.3g	30%
Total Sugars 8g	
Protein 8.5g	
Vitamin D 0mcg	0%
Calcium 52mg	4%
Iron 4mg	24%
Potassium 668mg	14%

*The % Daily Value (DV) tells you how much a nutrient in a food serving contributes to a daily diet. 2,000 calorie a day is used for general nutrition advice.

Recipe analyzed by verywell

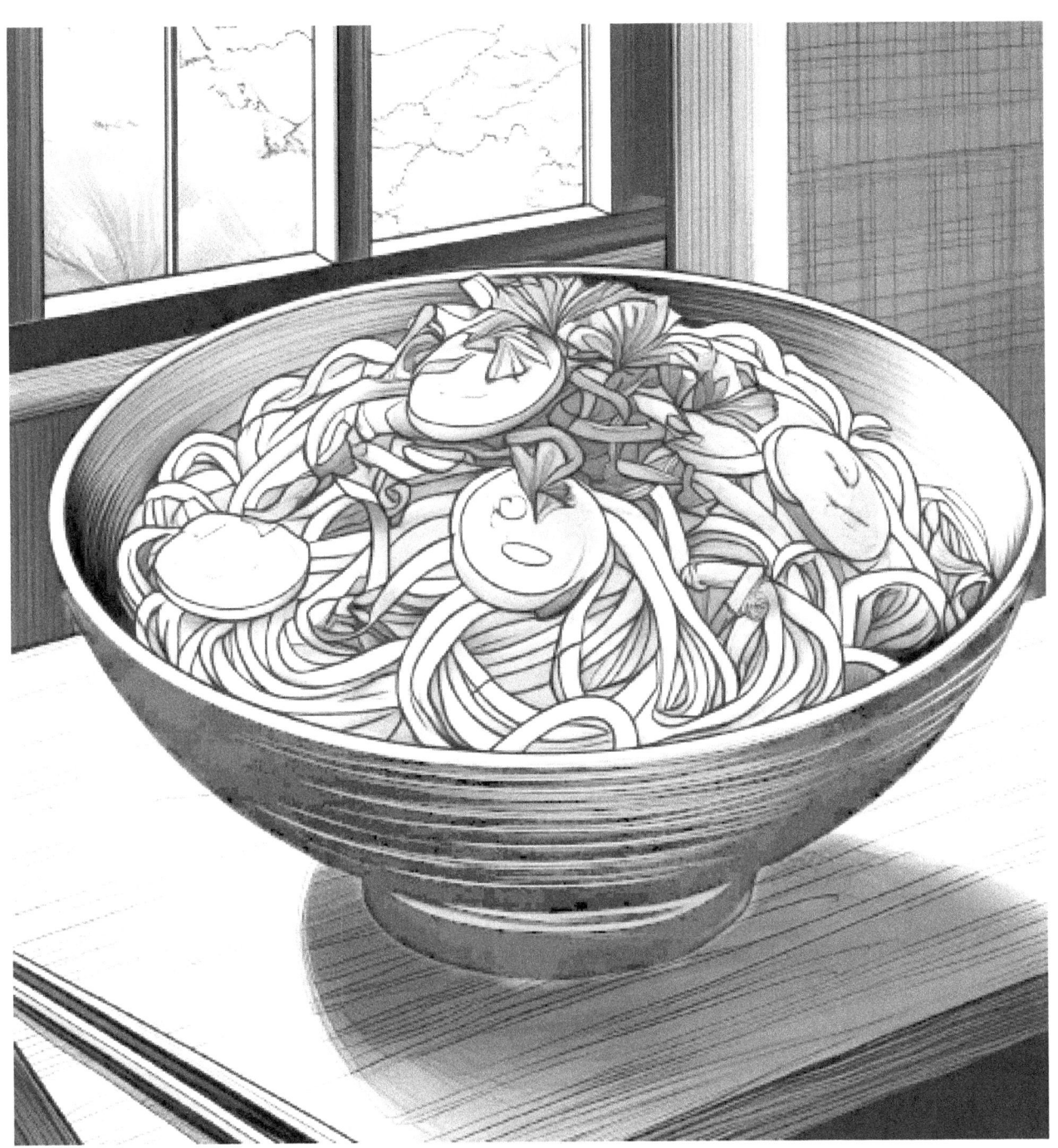

Ch 5: Entrees : Manchurian Noodles

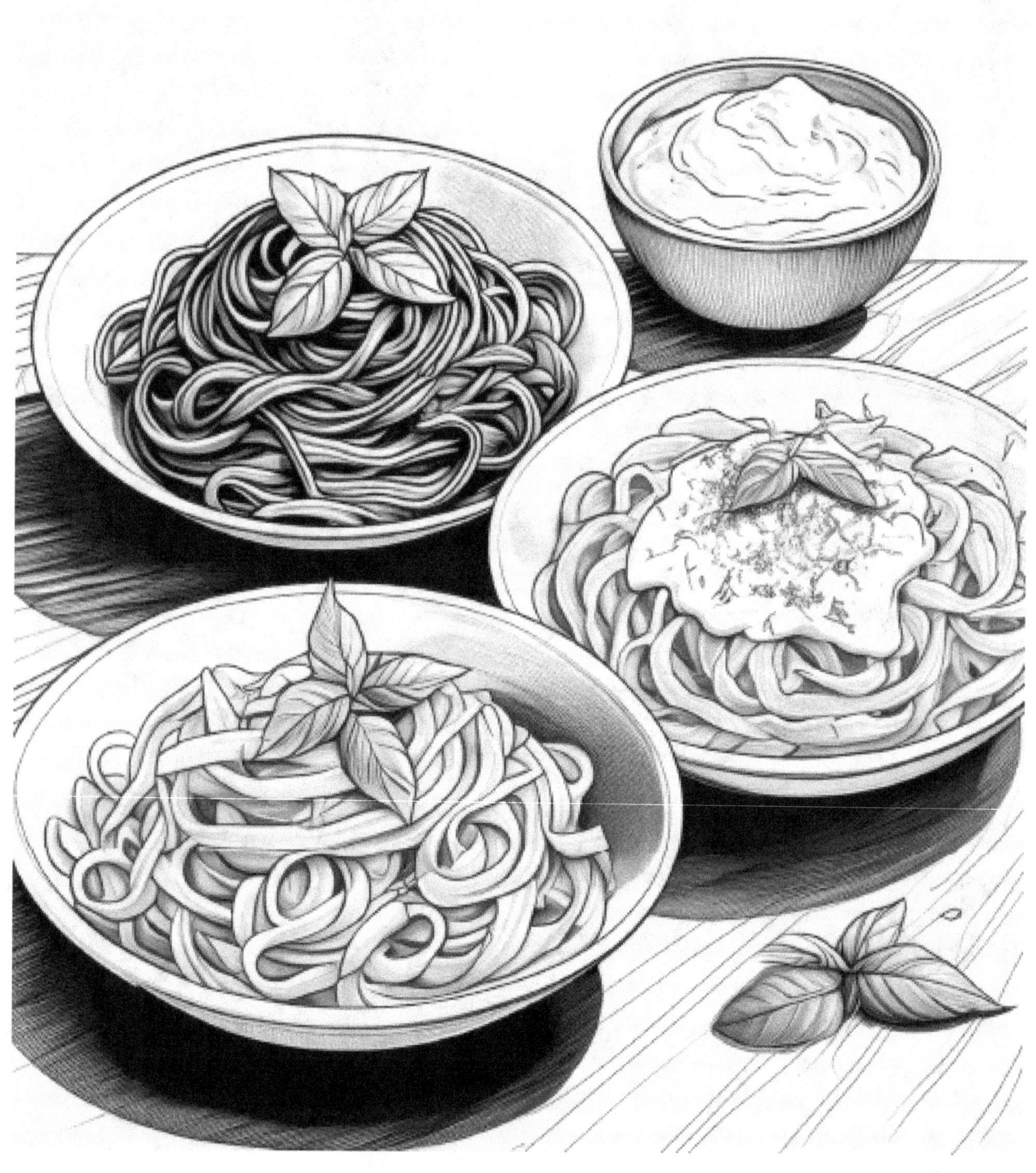

Ch 5: Entrees : Pastas & Sauces

Pastas
(Red Sauce, Creamy Alfredo, Pesto)

Explore three delightful pasta dishes with our sauces. For Red Sauce, cook pasta al dente, save some water, and sauté garlic and onion before adding tomatoes. Mix pasta with the sauce, using reserved water for consistency, and garnish with olive oil and herbs. For Creamy Alfredo, cook pasta al dente, strain, and mix with our hemp Alfredo sauce until creamy. Serve immediately for a rich, indulgent meal. For Pesto, cook pasta al dente, strain, and combine with our homemade pesto sauce. Serve warm or cool, garnished with cherry tomatoes and fresh herbs. These versatile recipes celebrate traditional flavors with a modern twist, perfect for any occasion. Minimalist and delicious.

Red Sauce

There are a few ways to cook your favorite pasta in red sauce. With the exposure to social media, you may have seen them. Here I utilize a more traditional approach.

1. In a pot, boil water adding a neutral oil and salt. Cook pasta al dente saving some of the water.
2. In a separate pan, lightly oil your pan. Add minced garlic and diced onion. Cook until onions are tender without burning the garlic. Add canned tomatoes and warm.
3. Last, using tongs, add cooked pasta to pan and coat with sauce. Add some of the reserved pasta water, heating the pan to serve hot. Garnish with a drizzle of olive oil and herbs.

Creamy Alfredo

1. In a large pan, boil water adding a neutral oil and salt. Cook pasta al dente and strain being sure to reserve some of the water.
2. Add hemp Alfredo sauce from the sauces section of this book.
3. Cook on medium heat until pasta is fully coated and sauce is warm with a creamy consistency. Serve immediately.

Pesto (Hot or Cold)

1. In a large pan, boil water adding a neutral oil and salt. Cook pasta al dente and strain being sure to reserve some of the water.
2. Add Pesto utilizing the Pesto recipe from the sauces section of this book. Warm and serve or serve cool. Garnish with halved cherry tomatoes and fresh herbs.

Nutrition Facts

Serving size: 1/2 Cup
Servings: 7

Amount per serving
Calories 380

	% Daily Value*
Total Fat 3g	4%
Saturated Fat 0g	0%
Cholesterol 0mg	0%
Sodium 0mg	0%
Total Carbohydrate 80g	29%
Dietary Fiber 10g	36%
Total Sugars 8g	
Protein 16g	
Vitamin D 0mcg	0%
Calcium 0mg	0%
Iron 4mg	20%
Potassium 440mg	9%

*The % Daily Value (DV) tells you how much a nutrient in a food serving contributes to a daily diet. 2,000 calorie a day is used for general nutrition advice.

Recipe analyzed by **well**

Crab Cake
(Lions Mane Mushroom)

Lion's Mane Mushroom is a culinary treasure with roots in traditional Asian medicine and cuisine, now embraced in modern American kitchens for its crab-like texture and seafood flavor. This recipe blends shredded Lion's Mane with diced onion, seasoned and panko bread crumbs, Old Bay seasoning, vegan mayo, Dijon mustard, and nori flakes for a touch of oceanic umami. Bound with an egg replacement, these ingredients create a delicious plant-based patty or addition to any meal. Lion's Mane Mushroom showcases the innovative spirit of plant-based cooking, transforming traditional ingredients into contemporary delights that appeal to both vegan enthusiasts and those seeking healthier eating options.

Ingredients

- 1 lb lion's mane mushroom, shredded
- 1/4 Cup finely diced onion
- 1/4 Cup Seasoned Bread Crumbs
- 1/4 Cup Panko Bread Crumbs
- 1 Tbsp Old Bay
- 2 Tbsp Vegan Mayonnaise
- 1/2 Tbsp Dijon mustard
- 1 Tbsp Powered Nori or Nori Flakes
- The equivalent of 1 Egg replacement

Instructions

1. Heat a large skillet over low heat (starting with low heat is very important). Once pan is warm add in about a tablespoon of oil and lion's mane to the pan.
2. Cook lion's mane about 10 minutes, stirring occasionally until tender and cooked through.
3. Sprinkle over 1/2 of the Old Bay and cook mushrooms 1 minute longer.
4. Transfer lion's mane to a large mixing bowl and let cool.
5. In the same pan increase heat to medium and add in a little more oil and onions to the pan.
6. Sprinkle lightly with salt. Cook onions, stirring occasionally until translucent. Turn off heat and add onions to bowl with lions mane and let cool.
7. Add remaining Old Bay, nori powder/flakes, breadcrumbs, mayo, dijon mustard, a pinch of pepper with the lions main and onions. Stir gently.
8. Add in egg replacement and stir gently to combine. Cover mixture and chill in refrigerator for at least 1 hour.
9. Portion crab cakes and place on lined baking sheet. Gently shape, being sure not to over flatten.
10. Lastly, Heat oil in a large pan over medium heat. Once pan is hot add vegan butter pan. Arrange crab cakes in hot pan 1-2 inches apart. Fry each side until golden brown.

Nutrition Facts

Serving size: 2 Crab Cakes
Servings: 8

Amount per serving

Calories 54

	% Daily Value*
Total Fat 2.7g	3%
Saturated Fat 0.3g	2%
Cholesterol 0mg	0%
Sodium 3498mg	152%
Total Carbohydrate 5.4g	2%
Dietary Fiber 0.5g	2%
Total Sugars 0.4g	
Protein 1.2g	
Vitamin D 0mcg	0%
Calcium 11mg	1%
Iron 0mg	2%
Potassium 23mg	0%

*The % Daily Value (DV) tells you how much a nutrient in a food serving contributes to a daily diet. 2,000 calorie a day is used for general nutrition advice.

Recipe analyzed by verywell

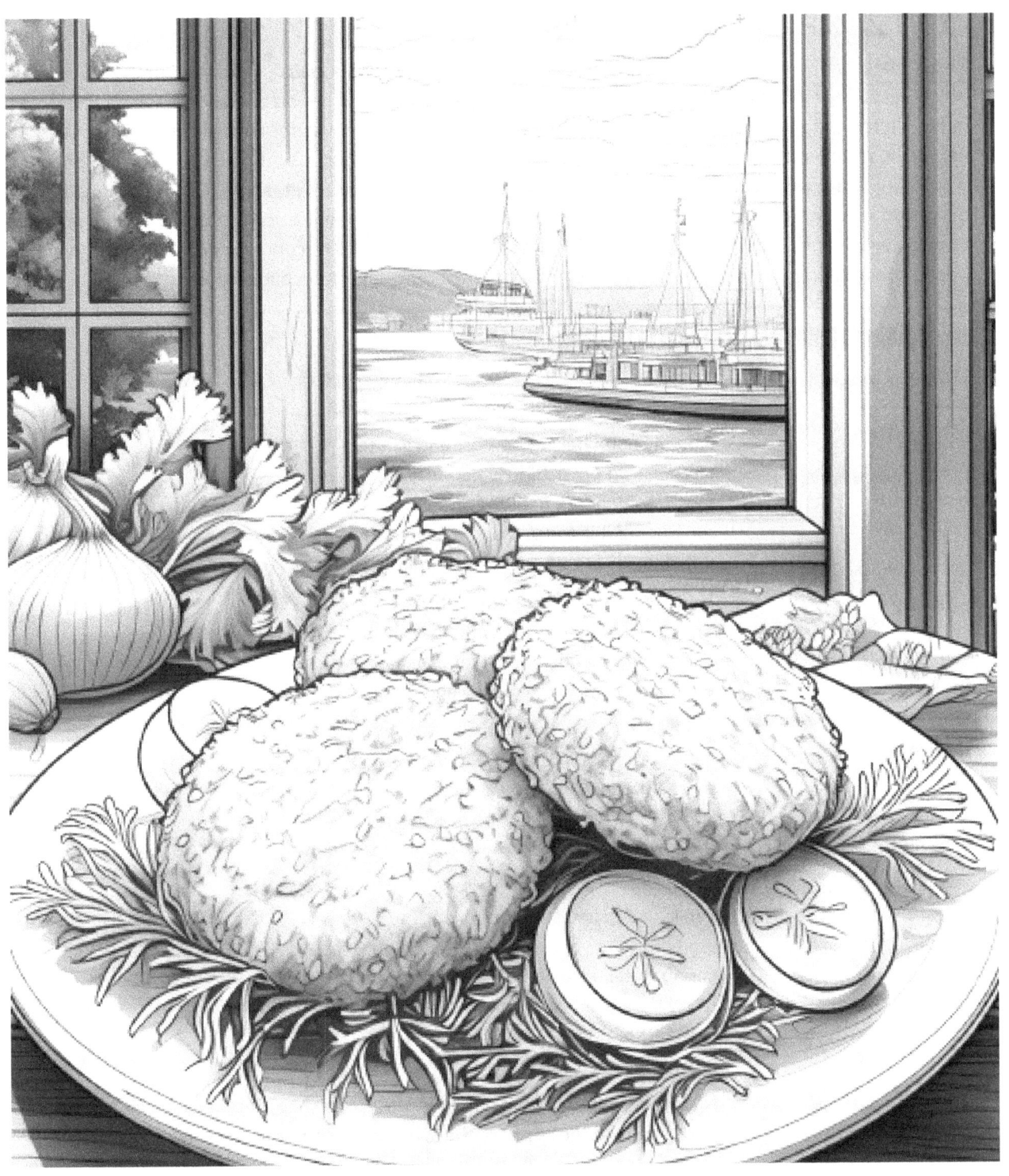

Ch 5: Entrees : Crab Cake

Pizza / Flatbread

Pizza/ Flatbread with Spelt Crust and Brazil Nut Cheese reimagines a classic favorite with nutritious, plant-based ingredients. This recipe pays homage to the rich tradition of pizza-making, which has evolved in the United States from its Italian immigrant roots to a versatile canvas for culinary creativity. Our version features a wholesome spelt flour crust, bringing a nutty, robust flavor and added health benefits. Topped with a creamy Brazil nut cheese, made with key lime juice, sea salt, and a hint of cayenne for a delightful kick, this dish celebrates the innovative spirit of modern vegan cuisine. Perfect for those looking to enjoy a guilt-free indulgence, this pizza/flatbread is a testament to the endless possibilities of plant-based cooking, transforming traditional recipes into nutritious, flavorful masterpieces.

Ingredients (Dough)

- 1/2 Cup Warm Water
- 1 Tsp Agave
- 1 Tsp Avocado Oil
- 1 1/2 cups Spelt Flour
- 1 1/2 Tsp Baking Powder
- 1/4 Tsp Sea Salt
- 2-3 Tbsp Sauce

Ingredients (Cheese)

- 1 lb. Brazil Nuts*
- 1/2 of a Key Lime
- 2 Tsp Sea Salt
- 1 Tsp Onion Powder
- 1/2 Tsp Cayenne
- 1 1/2 Cup Hemp Milk
- 1 1/2 Cup Spring Water
- 2 Tsp Avocado Oil

*It is best to soak the Brazil nuts overnight.

Instructions

1. In a large bowl add the warm water, agave and avocado oil. Mix until the agave is dissolved.

2. Add the flour, baking powder and salt to a large mixing bowl. Slowly add wet ingredients mixing with a fork until the dough comes together (If it is too dry, add a little more water until it holds together to form a ball).

3. Flour your counter and turn out the dough. Knead, sprinkling lightly with flour so it doesn't stick to your hands. Knead for 3-4 minutes until the dough is no longer sticky and is smooth.

4. Coat the mixing bowl with a little oil and put the dough back in the bowl and cover with a towel. Place in a warm place (an oven with the light on has been said to be perfect) to allow the dough to rest after kneading. Remove from the oven after 30 minutes.

5. While dough is resting, add all of your cheese ingredients to your blender, excluding the spring water. Adding only 1/2 cup of water, blend the ingredients together for 2 minutes. Continue to add 1/2 cup of water and blend until the desired consistency is reached.

6. Next press out dough on a floured surface to shape. Add any of the 3 sauces (red, creamy or pesto) from the sauces section of this book, along with veggies and any topping you want (Brazil nut cheese is a great addition).*

7. With the rack in the low position, bake at 450° for 15 to 20 minutes or until you get the desired texture of dough for your pizzas.

Nutrition Facts

Serving size: 2 Slices
Servings: 8

Amount per serving

Calories   163

	% Daily Value*
Total Fat 2.9g	4%
Saturated Fat 0.6g	3%
Cholesterol 0mg	0%
Sodium 293mg	13%
Total Carbohydrate 32.2g	12%
Dietary Fiber 4.2g	15%
Total Sugars 14.1g	
Protein 3.3g	
Vitamin D 0mcg	0%
Calcium 30mg	2%
Iron 1mg	6%
Potassium 199mg	4%

*The % Daily Value (DV) tells you how much a nutrient in a food serving contributes to a daily diet. 2,000 calorie a day is used for general nutrition advice.

Recipe analyzed by verywell

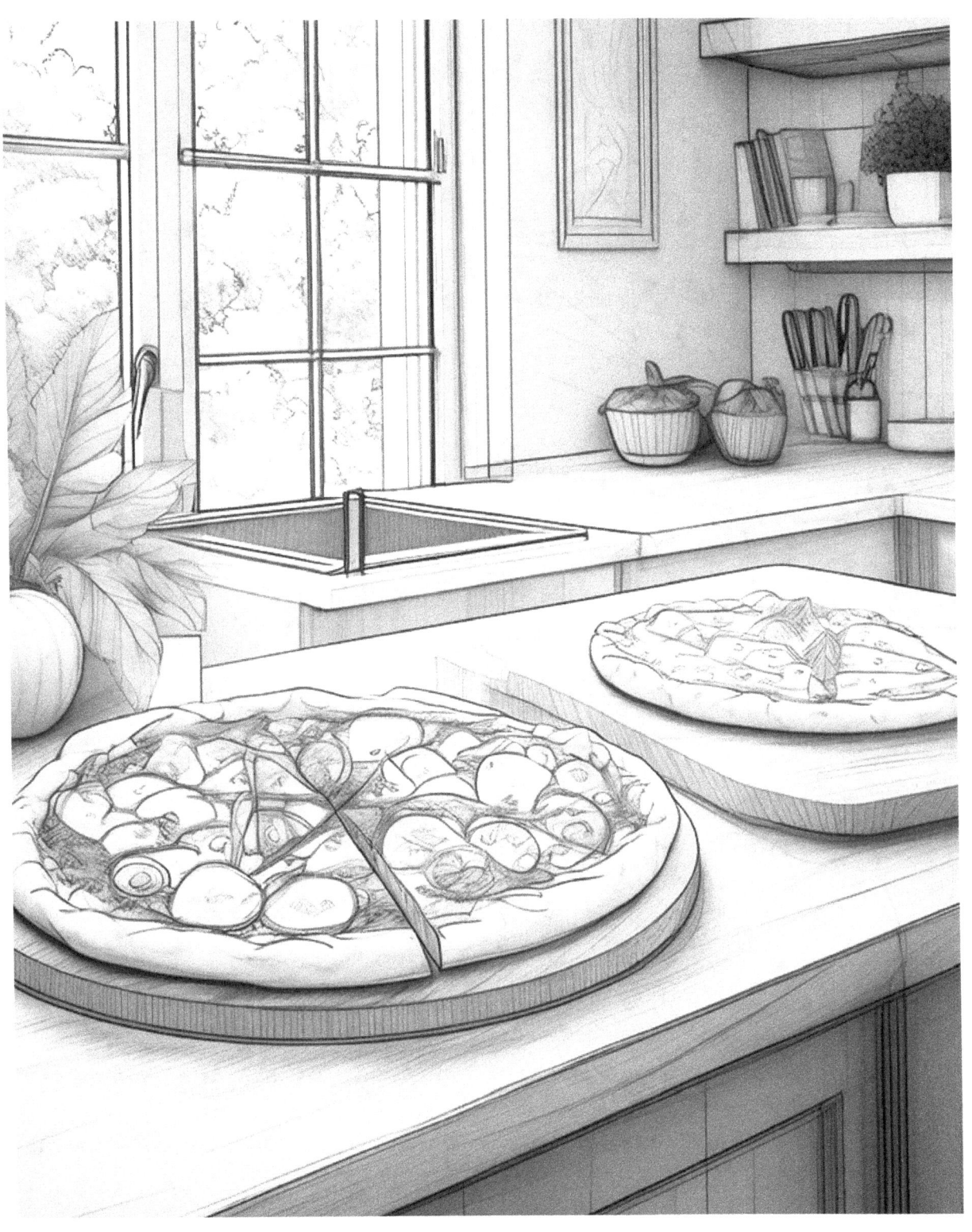

59

Ch 5: Entrees : Pizza / Flatbread

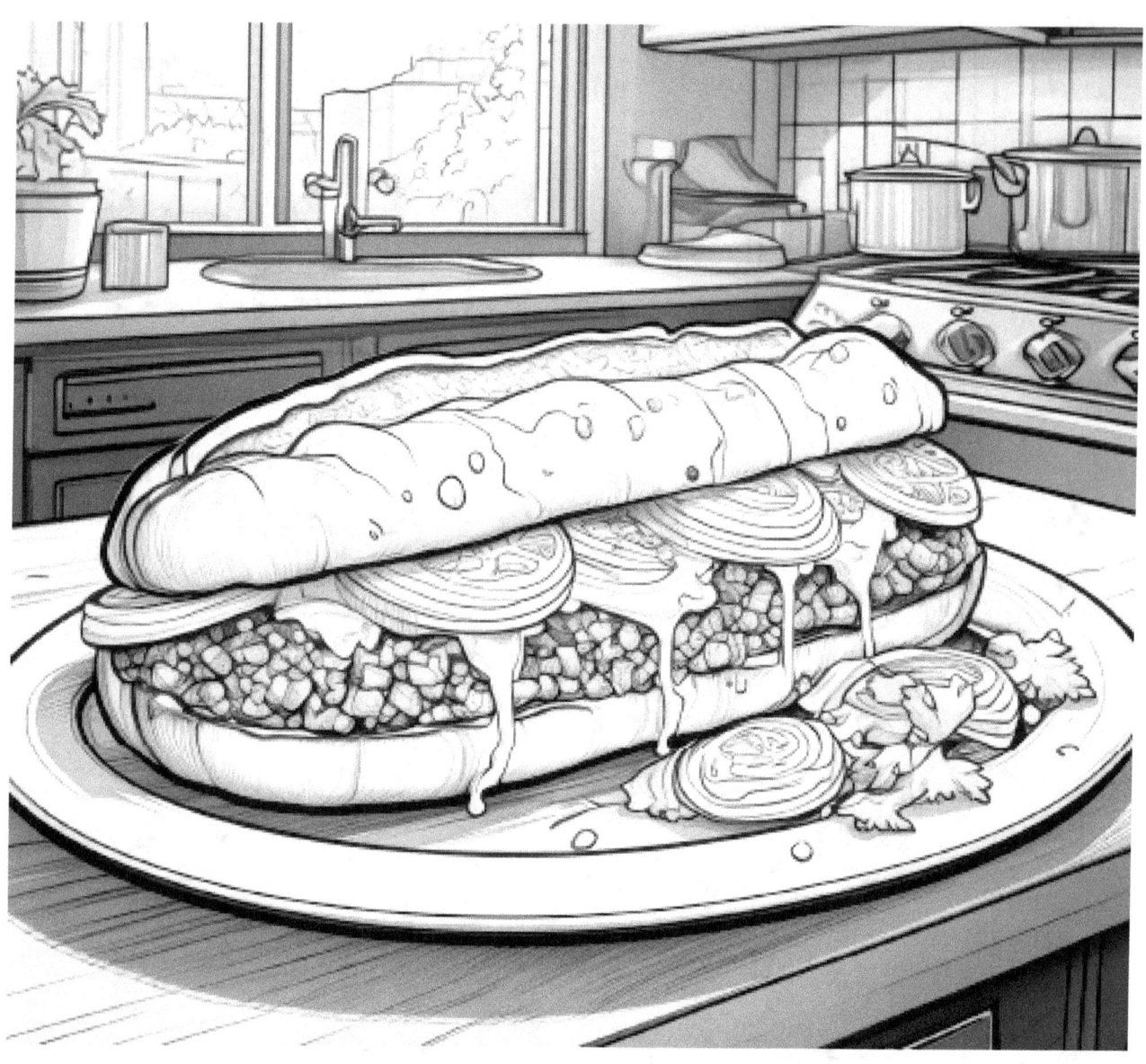

Walnuts and Mushrooms can be substituted with your favorite beef like meat replacement if you are allergic to walnuts or have a hard time digesting mushrooms.

Research says boiling mushrooms prior to using them in recipes can potentially make them more meat like and may assist with digesting them.

Soak walnuts for at least 12 hours before making this recipe. A lot of people suggest 24 hours to make sure they are soft.

Ch 5: Entrees : Chopped Cheese

Chopped Cheese

Chopped Cheese is a flavorful, plant-based take on a classic American sandwich, known for its roots in New York City's bodega culture. This recipe substitutes the traditional beef with a savory mixture of raw walnuts and Baby Bella mushrooms, offering a hearty and satisfying texture. Combined with sweet onion, garlic, and a blend of spices including black pepper, garlic powder, onion powder, and Adobo, the filling is brought to life with the addition of Better Than Bouillon no-beef base. Perfect for sandwiches or wraps, this Chopped Cheese honors the innovative spirit of Moorish American cuisine, transforming beloved comfort foods into healthy, plant-based delights. Enjoy a taste of culinary history with a modern twist, making this dish both nostalgic and nutritious.

Ingredients

- 1 Cup Raw Walnuts
- 1 Cup Baby Bella Mushrooms
- 1 Sweet Onion
- 2 Cloves Garlic
- 1 Tsp Better Than Bouillon no-beef base
- 1 Tbsp Black Pepper
- 1 Tbsp Garlic Powder
- 1 Tbsp Onion Powder
- 1 Tbsp Adobo

Instructions

1. In a food processor, combine walnuts, mushrooms, 1/2 the onion & garlic and pulse to create a minced ground texture.
2. In a hot skillet add avocado oil to prevent sticking. Sauté the other half of the onion and garlic, followed by the walnut and mushroom mixture.
3. Add No-Beef Bouillon, garlic powder, onion powder, adobo, and black pepper. Mix well to combine.
4. Lastly add your favorite vegan American cheese, chop and mix until the cheese is melted and fully incorporated into the walnut and mushroom mixture.
5. Serve on your favorite sub roll or in a wrap with your favorite vegan mayonnaise, ketchup, lettuce, tomatoes and burro fries on the side.

Nutrition Facts — Walnut Meat

Serving size: 1 Cup
Servings: 3

Amount per serving
Calories 315

	% Daily Value*
Total Fat 24.8g	32%
Saturated Fat 1.4g	7%
Cholesterol 0mg	0%
Sodium 352mg	15%
Total Carbohydrate 17.3g	6%
Dietary Fiber 5.2g	18%
Total Sugars 4.1g	
Protein 12.8g	
Vitamin D 0mcg	0%
Calcium 67mg	5%
Iron 2mg	13%
Potassium 514mg	11%

*The % Daily Value (DV) tells you how much a nutrient in a food serving contributes to a daily diet. 2,000 calorie a day is used for general nutrition advice.

Recipe analyzed by **well**

Nutrition Facts — "Cheese"

Serving size: 2 Slices
Servings: 8

Amount per serving
Calories 90

	% Daily Value*
Total Fat 8.2g	11%
Saturated Fat 1.7g	8%
Cholesterol 0mg	0%
Sodium 145mg	6%
Total Carbohydrate 3.5g	1%
Dietary Fiber 2.5g	9%
Total Sugars 0.4g	
Protein 1.6g	
Vitamin D 0mcg	1%
Calcium 67mg	5%
Iron 1mg	3%
Potassium 175mg	4%

*The % Daily Value (DV) tells you how much a nutrient in a food serving contributes to a daily diet. 2,000 calorie a day is used for general nutrition advice.

Recipe analyzed by **well**

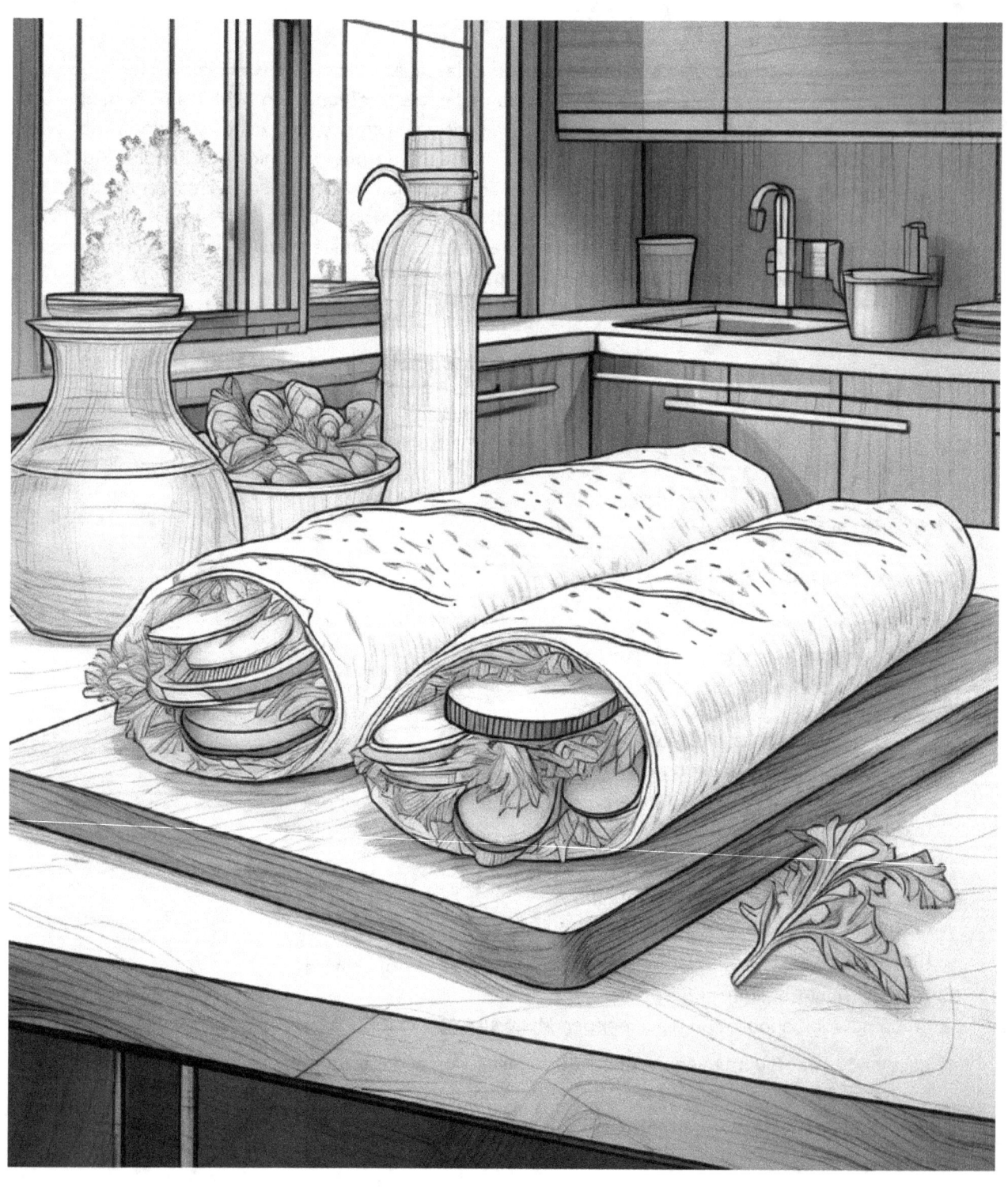

Ch 5: Entrees : Wraps/ Sandwiches

Wraps / Sandwiches
(Veggie Salads, Smoked Zucchini, etc)

Wraps and Sandwiches with Smoked Zucchini bring a delightful, plant-based twist to classic favorites. This recipe features marinated zucchini strips, seasoned with a blend of Adobo, Sazon, garlic powder, onion powder, liquid smoke, smoked paprika, and Italian herbs, creating a rich, smoky flavor. Perfectly sautéed, these zucchini strips serve as an innovative, flavorful meat replacement. Use them hot or cold in wraps or on sandwich rolls, paired with vegan mayonnaise, cheese, lettuce, tomato, and onions. This dish transforms simple vegetables into hearty, satisfying meals that honor tradition while embracing modern, plant-based eating.

Ingredients

- 1 Large Zucchini
- 1 Tbsp Avocado Oil
- 1 Tbsp Adobo
- 1 Packet Sazon
- 1 Tbsp Garlic Powder
- 1 Tbsp Onion Powder
- 1 Tbsp Liquid Smoke
- 1/2 Tbsp Smoked Paprika
- 2 Tbsp Italian Herb Blend

Instructions

1. In a large bowl or dish slice zucchini the long way to make strips. I use a peeler for consistency.
2. Next add the oil and all of the seasoning ingredients to a separate bowl and mix well to make a marinade.
3. Pour marinade over zucchini and mix well ensuring all of the strips are evenly coated.
4. Marinate for one hour or longer.
5. In a large skillet or flat top heat oil and sauté on medium heat until tender.
6. Serve hot or cold as a smoked meat replacement in a wrap or on your favorite sandwich roll with vegan mayonnaise, cheese, lettuce, tomato, and onions.

Nutrition Facts

Serving size: 4 Slices
Servings: 8

Amount per serving
Calories   31

	% Daily Value*
Total Fat 1.9g	2%
Saturated Fat 0.3g	1%
Cholesterol 0mg	0%
Sodium 155mg	7%
Total Carbohydrate 3.3g	1%
Dietary Fiber 0.8g	3%
Total Sugars 1.4g	
Protein 0.8g	
Vitamin D 0mcg	0%
Calcium 11mg	1%
Iron 0mg	2%
Potassium 136mg	3%

*The % Daily Value (DV) tells you how much a nutrient in a food serving contributes to a daily diet. 2,000 calorie a day is used for general nutrition advice.

Recipe analyzed by **well**

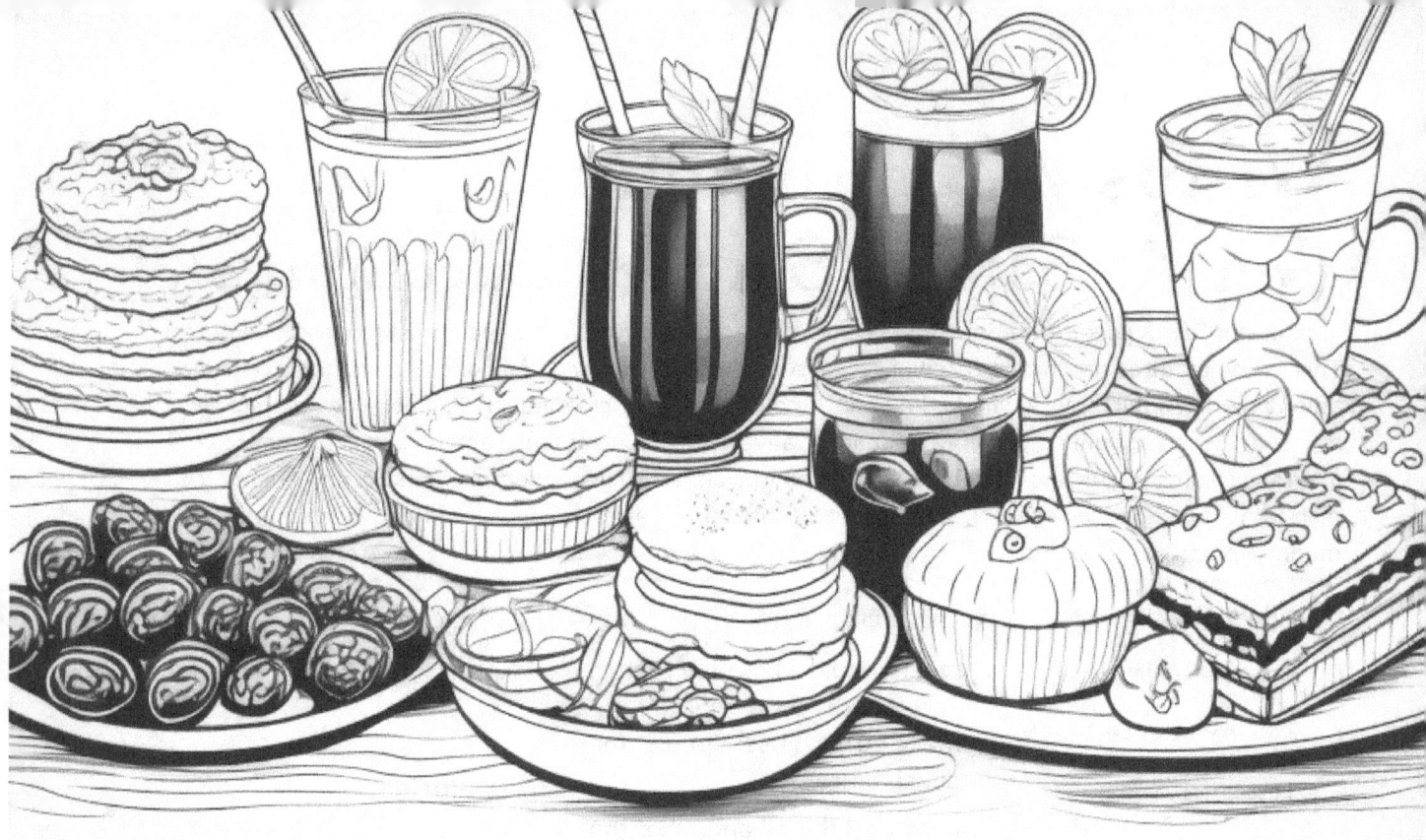

6.
SIPS
AND
SWEETS

In this chapter, we explore a variety of refreshing drinks and delightful treats that celebrate the rich culinary traditions of the Americas. From the tangy Tamarindo and vibrant Hibiscus (Sorrel) drinks to nutrient-packed Sea Moss Smoothies and classic Limeade, each beverage offers a unique taste experience rooted in natural ingredients. The Peanut Butter Dates combine the creamy richness of peanut butter with the natural sweetness of dates, providing a simple yet indulgent snack. The Banana Bread, enriched with spelt, chickpea, and coconut flours, brings a nutritious twist to a beloved classic. For a raw, plant-based dessert, the Strawberry Cheesecake Donuts offer a delicious blend of fresh strawberries and creamy walnuts. These recipes highlight the harmony of traditional flavors and modern tastes, providing a delightful way to enjoy wholesome, plant-based ingredients.

Tamarindo

Tamarindo, a beverage rooted in the rich culinary traditions of the Americas, embodies a fusion of indigenous flavors and contemporary tastes. This refreshing drink, made from tamarind fruit, key limes, and agave, harkens back to the ancient civilizations that enjoyed tamarind for its tangy, invigorating properties. Traditionally enjoyed across Latin America, tamarindo captures the essence of cultural heritage while offering a vibrant, thirst-quenching experience. Perfect for hot days or festive occasions, this drink not only refreshes but also connects us to the historical and culinary tapestry of the Americas.

Ingredients

- 1 Lb Fresh Tamarind
- 5 Key Limes
- 1/2 - 1 Cup Agave
- 1 Gallon of Spring Water

Instructions

1. Peel tamarind fruit from pods. In a large pot boil 1/2 of the water. Put peeled fruit in pot. Turn off heat and mash (I use a whisk), separating the fruit from the seeds.
2. Strain into a large bowl.
3. Use the other 1/2 of the water to rinse left over fruit while mashing through the strainer to ensure all of the remaining fruit is separated from the seeds.
4. Once you get the seeds completely separated, transfer the juice to a bottle (using a funnel), juice key limes, sweeten with agave and enjoy.

Nutrition Facts

Serving size: 1 Cup
Servings: 12

Amount per serving

Calories   **44**

% Daily Value*

Total Fat 0.1g	0%
Saturated Fat 0g	0%
Cholesterol 0mg	0%
Sodium 3mg	0%
Total Carbohydrate 12.8g	5%
Dietary Fiber 1.8g	6%
Total Sugars 8.5g	
Protein 0.5g	
Vitamin D 0mcg	0%
Calcium 20mg	2%
Iron 0mg	3%
Potassium 95mg	2%

*The % Daily Value (DV) tells you how much a nutrient in a food serving contributes to a daily diet. 2,000 calorie a day is used for general nutrition advice.

Recipe analyzed by **well**

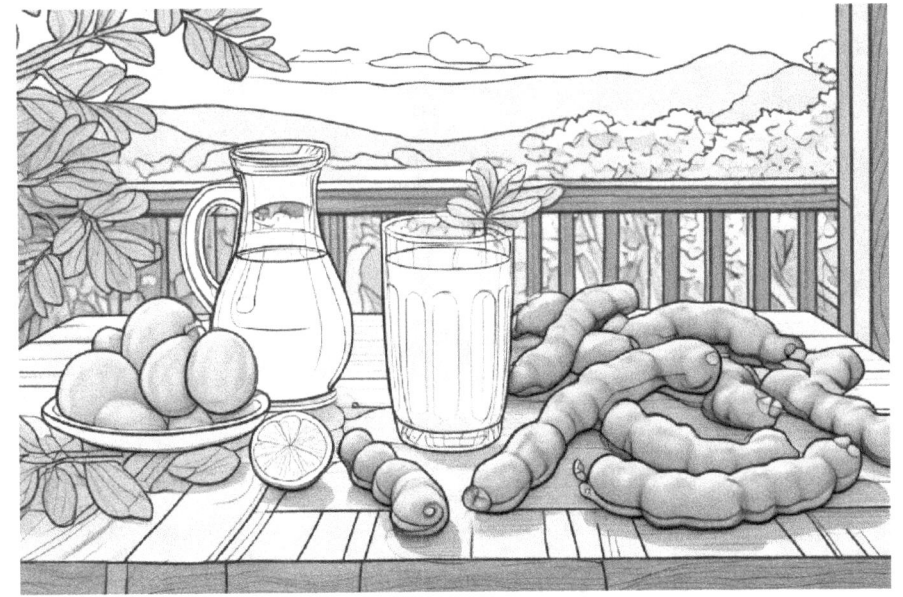

Ch 6: Sips & Sweets : Tamarindo

Hibiscus (Sorrel)

Hibiscus (Sorrel) is a vibrant, tangy drink with deep roots in the culinary traditions of the Americas. Combining dried hibiscus flowers, fresh ginger, cloves, and allspice, this refreshing beverage is sweetened with agave and infused with spring water. Historically enjoyed throughout the Caribbean and Central America, Sorrel offers a delightful balance of tartness and spice, making it a perfect, rejuvenating treat. This drink captures the essence of wholesome, natural ingredients, offering a taste that's both nostalgic and invigorating. Enjoy this flavorful beverage as a unique addition to your plant-based sips, celebrating the harmony of traditional flavors and modern tastes.

Ingredients

- 3 Cups Dried Hibiscus
- 1 LB Fresh Ginger
- 12 Cloves
- 9 Allspice Berries
- 1 1/2 Cups Agave
- 1 Gallon Spring Water

Instructions

1. Start by grating your ginger and smashing the allspice (unless you're using powder).
2. In a large pot bring 12 cups of water to a boil. Add hibiscus, grated ginger, cloves, and allspice to the pot and boil for about 10 minutes.
3. Remove from heat and let cool.
4. Transfer to an airtight container and steep for 48 hours (minimum overnight).
5. Strain in a large bowl to separate the solids ensuring you retain as much of the liquid as possible. Bottle, sweeten, and serve.

Nutrition Facts

Serving size: 1 Cup
Servings: 12

Amount per serving

Calories 252

% Daily Value*

Total Fat 8.5g	11%
Saturated Fat 2.2g	11%
Cholesterol 0mg	0%
Sodium 160mg	7%
Total Carbohydrate 63.9g	23%
Dietary Fiber 16.8g	60%
Total Sugars 8.9g	
Protein 4.9g	
Vitamin D 0mcg	0%
Calcium 496mg	38%
Iron 5mg	29%
Potassium 783mg	17%

*The % Daily Value (DV) tells you how much a nutrient in a food serving contributes to a daily diet. 2,000 calorie a day is used for general nutrition advice.

Recipe analyzed by verywell

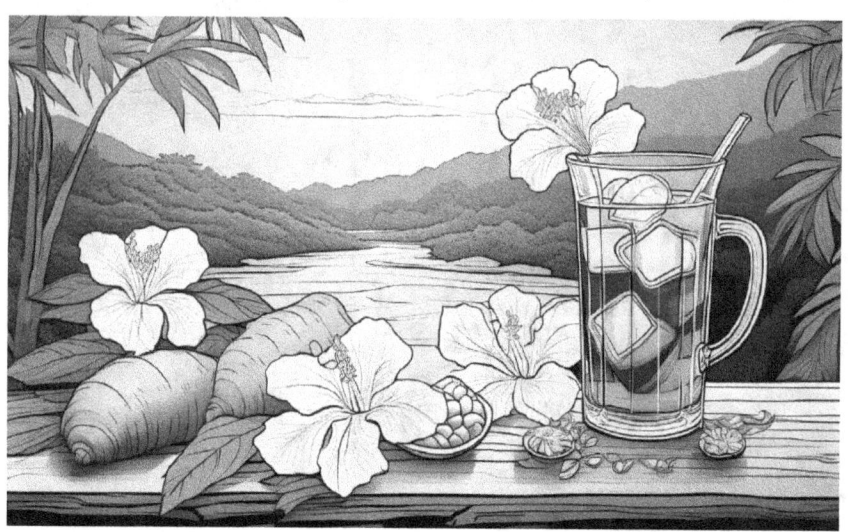

Limeade

Limeade, a refreshing drink with deep roots in the Americas, captures the vibrant flavors of key limes and the natural sweetness of agave. Historically, limes have been a staple in various cultures, prized for their refreshing taste and health benefits. This simple yet invigorating beverage combines freshly squeezed lime juice with spring water, offering a perfect balance of tart and sweet. Limeade evokes the essence of sunny days and shared moments, providing a delicious way to stay hydrated and enjoy the natural bounty. This timeless classic is perfect for any occasion, celebrating the simplicity and richness of natural ingredients.

Ingredients

- 24 Key Limes
- 1-2 Cups Agave
- 1 Gallon Spring Water

Step 1

1. Cut lime and juice them into a pitcher.
2. Add spring water and sweeten.

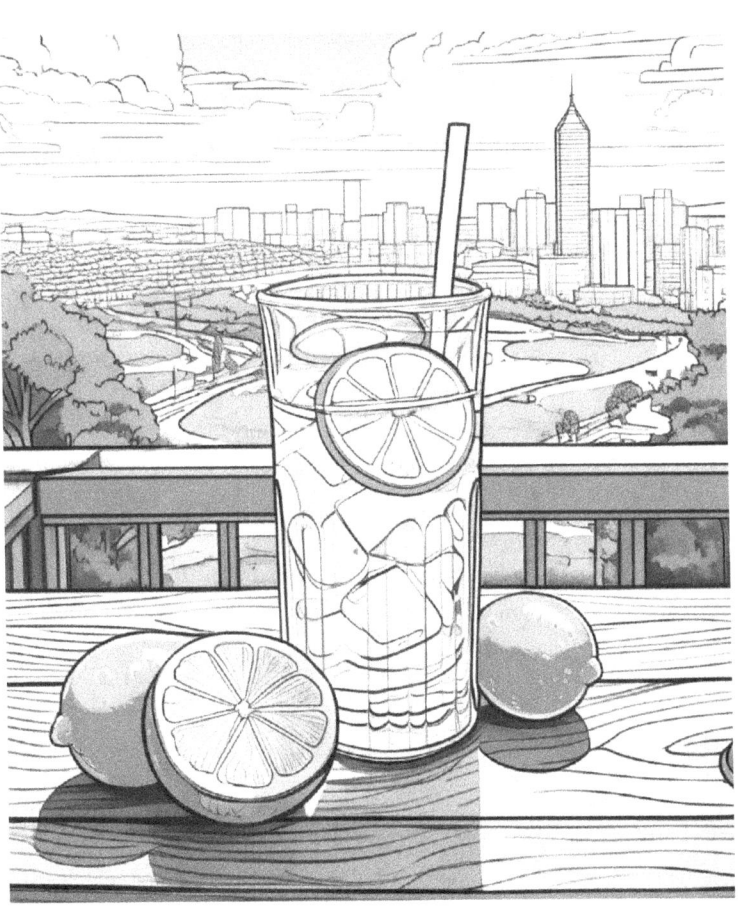

Nutrition Facts

Serving size: 1 Cup
Servings: 12

Amount per serving

Calories 88

	% Daily Value*
Total Fat 0g	0%
Saturated Fat 0g	0%
Cholesterol 0mg	0%
Sodium 0mg	0%
Total Carbohydrate 26.7g	10%
Dietary Fiber 4.8g	17%
Total Sugars 11.9g	
Protein 0g	
Vitamin D 0mcg	0%
Calcium 0mg	0%
Iron 0mg	0%
Potassium 0mg	0%

*The % Daily Value (DV) tells you how much a nutrient in a food serving contributes to a daily diet. 2,000 calorie a day is used for general nutrition advice.

Recipe analyzed by **well**

Ch 6: Sips & Sweets : Limeade

Seamoss Smoothies

Sea moss smoothies are a nod to the rich, natural ingredients of the Americas, blending traditional knowledge with modern tastes. These smoothies, featuring tropical fruits like mango, papaya, and berries, are infused with nutrient-dense sea moss, revered for its health benefits. Each variation offers a unique, refreshing taste, from the tangy burst of strawberry lime to the sweet medley of mixed berries, and the tropical harmony of mango and papaya. Embracing the bounty of the Americas, these smoothies are a delicious and nourishing way to enjoy the diverse flavors and benefits of sea moss.

Strawberry Lime:

- 2 Cups Frozen Strawberries
- 2 Cups Fresh Limeade
- 3 Tbsp Seamoss

Add all ingredients to blender and blend until smooth.

Mixed Berry (Raspberry, Blackberry, Blueberry, Strawberry)

- 3 Cups Frozen Berry Blend
- 2 Cups Frozen Strawberries
- 1 Cup Frozen Blueberries
- 2 Cups Grape Juice
- 1 Cup Spring Water
- 3 Tbsp Seamoss

Add all ingredients to blender and blend until smooth.

Tropical (Mango + Papaya)

- 2 Cups Frozen Mango
- 2 Fresh Mangoes
- 2 Cups Fresh Papaya
- 2 Cups Coconut Water
- 3 Tbsp Seamoss

1. Cut, peel and cube fresh mango and papaya.
2. Add all ingredients to blender and blend until smooth.

*Keep papaya seeds with fruit and include in your smoothies for their incredible benefits.

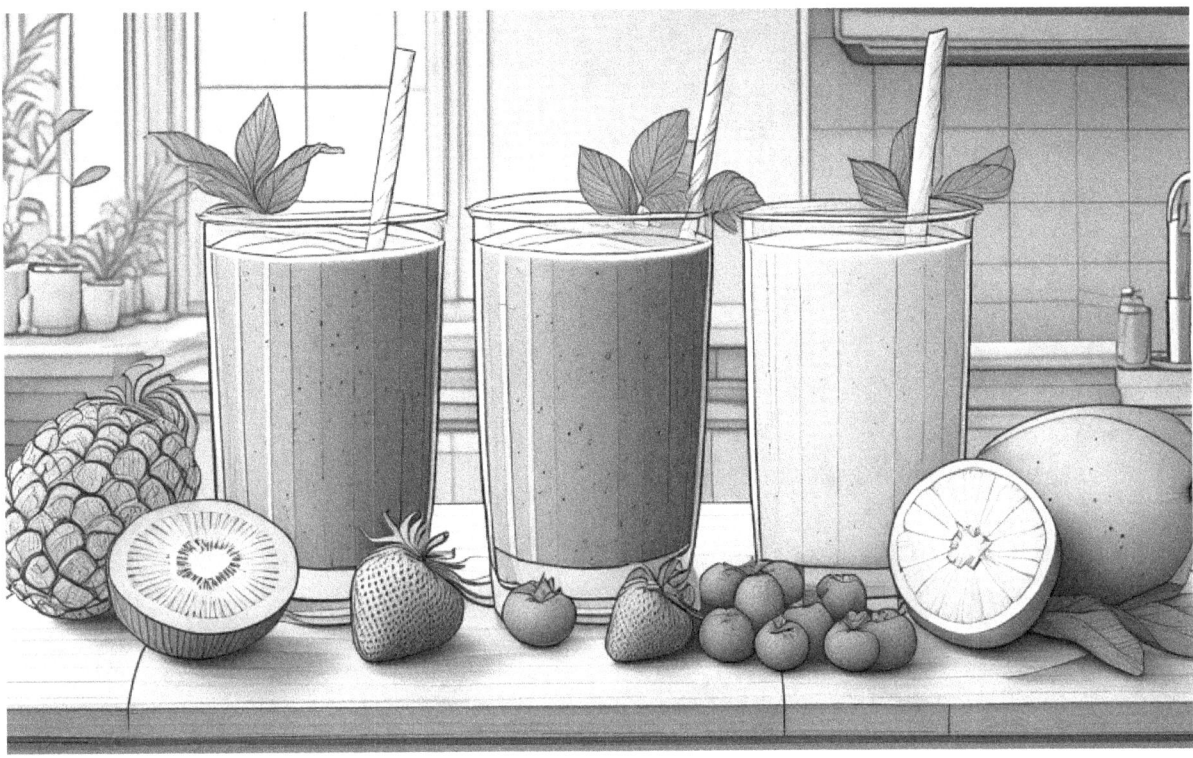

Strawberry Lime

Nutrition Facts

Serving size: 1 Cup
Servings: 3

Amount per serving
Calories   107

% Daily Value*

Total Fat 0g	0%
Saturated Fat 0g	0%
Cholesterol 0mg	0%
Sodium 10mg	0%
Total Carbohydrate 27g	10%
Dietary Fiber 1.5g	5%
Total Sugars 24g	
Protein 0.2g	
Vitamin D 0mcg	0%
Calcium 29mg	2%
Iron 1mg	7%
Potassium 50mg	1%

*The % Daily Value (DV) tells you how much a nutrient in a food serving contributes to a daily diet. 2,000 calorie a day is used for general nutrition advice.

Recipe analyzed by **well**

Mixed Berry

Nutrition Facts

Serving size: 1 Cup
Servings: 3

Amount per serving
Calories   178

% Daily Value*

Total Fat 0.7g	1%
Saturated Fat 0g	0%
Cholesterol 0mg	0%
Sodium 13mg	1%
Total Carbohydrate 44.2g	16%
Dietary Fiber 18.6g	66%
Total Sugars 21.8g	
Protein 1.8g	
Vitamin D 0mcg	0%
Calcium 41mg	3%
Iron 3mg	15%
Potassium 44mg	1%

*The % Daily Value (DV) tells you how much a nutrient in a food serving contributes to a daily diet. 2,000 calorie a day is used for general nutrition advice.

Recipe analyzed by **well**

Tropical

Nutrition Facts

Serving size: 1 Cup
Servings: 3

Amount per serving
Calories   271

% Daily Value*

Total Fat 1.5g	2%
Saturated Fat 0.6g	3%
Cholesterol 0mg	0%
Sodium 185mg	8%
Total Carbohydrate 67.2g	24%
Dietary Fiber 9.2g	33%
Total Sugars 56.4g	
Protein 3.6g	
Vitamin D 0mcg	0%
Calcium 90mg	7%
Iron 2mg	11%
Potassium 1105mg	24%

*The % Daily Value (DV) tells you how much a nutrient in a food serving contributes to a daily diet. 2,000 calorie a day is used for general nutrition advice.

Recipe analyzed by **well**

Ch 6: Sips & Sweets : Seamoss Smoothies

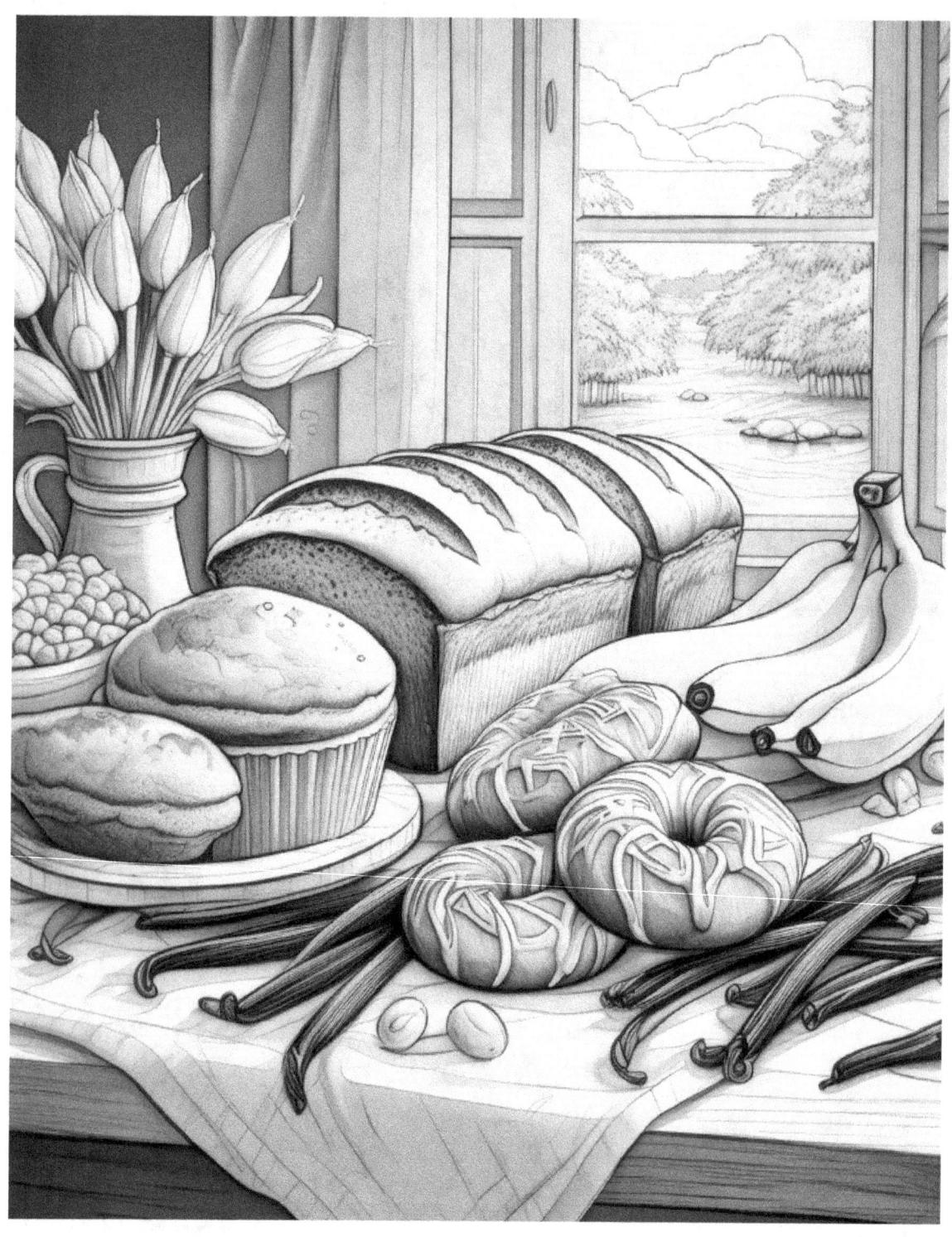

Ch 6: Sips & Sweets : Seamoss Smoothies

Banana Bread / Muffins / Donuts

Banana bread, a beloved classic, brings the comforting sweetness of ripe bananas into a moist, flavorful loaf. This recipe, enriched with spelt, chickpea, and coconut flours, offers a nutritious twist while maintaining the familiar, indulgent taste. Sweetened with agave and enhanced by the subtle tang of key lime and the richness of walnuts, this banana bread is a celebration of wholesome, natural ingredients. Perfect for breakfast or an afternoon treat, it embodies the simplicity and warmth of home baking. Enjoy this timeless favorite, reflecting a blend of tradition and innovation in every bite.

Ingredients

- 10 Baby Bananas or 5 Regular Bananas
- 1.5 Cups Spelt Flour
- 1/2 Cup Chickpea Flour
- 1/2 Cup Coconut Flour
- 3/4 Cup Agave
- 1 Tsp Sea Salt
- 2 Tsp Baking Soda
- 1 Tsp Pure Vanilla Extract
- 6 Tbsp Grapeseed Oil
- 1 Key Lime
- 1/2 Cup Hemp Milk
- 1/2 Cup Perrier
- 1 Cup Walnuts

Instructions

1. Add mashed bananas to wet ingredients then fold wet ingredients into dry ingredients
2. Preheat oven to 350. Bake in 8in bread pan for 55 minutes to 1 hour.

Nutrition Facts

Serving size: 1 - 2 Muffins
Servings: 8

Amount per serving

Calories   **445**

% Daily Value*

Total Fat 19.2g	25%
Saturated Fat 1.7g	9%
Cholesterol 0mg	0%
Sodium 233mg	10%
Total Carbohydrate 64.4g	23%
Dietary Fiber 11.5g	41%
Total Sugars 29.5g	
Protein 10.1g	
Vitamin D 0mcg	0%
Calcium 52mg	4%
Iron 3mg	15%
Potassium 282mg	6%

*The % Daily Value (DV) tells you how much a nutrient in a food serving contributes to a daily diet. 2,000 calorie a day is used for general nutrition advice.

Recipe analyzed by **well**

Raw Strawberry Cheesecake Donuts

Raw strawberry cheesecake donuts are a delightful fusion of fresh strawberries and creamy walnuts, offering a plant-based twist on a classic dessert. This recipe uses natural ingredients like dates, sea moss gel, and key lime to create a rich, flavorful filling and a nutty, crumbly crust. Perfectly balancing sweetness and tang, these raw treats are both indulgent and nutritious. Enjoy the vibrant flavors and smooth texture that make this raw strawberry cheesecake a standout addition to any dessert table, celebrating the simplicity and purity of whole, plant-based ingredients.

Filling

- 2 Cups Strawberries (1/2 Frozen)
- 1 Cup Walnuts
- 1 Key Lime
- 1/4 Tsp Salt
- 12 Dates
- 3 Tbsp Sea Moss Gel

Crust

- 1 Cup Walnuts
- 12 Dates
- 1/4 Tsp Salt

Topping

- 6 Large Strawberries
- 2 Tbsp Sea Moss Gel
- 1 Tsp Agave

Instructions

1. Start by adding crust ingredients to you food processor. Pulse until mixed well and a crumble is formed.
2. Add crumble to parchment lined spring form pan, press down to form crust.
3. Next, add 2 cups of strawberries to your blender. Blend until smooth. Then add walnuts, the juice of the key lime and salt. Blend until smooth.
4. Next, add dates and sea moss gel, blend until smooth once more.
5. Add strawberry mixture to the crust.
6. Add topping ingredients to blender and blend until smooth.
7. Last. add blended strawberry topping to the pan and evenly distribute.
8. Refrigerate or freeze for a few hours to set and then serve.

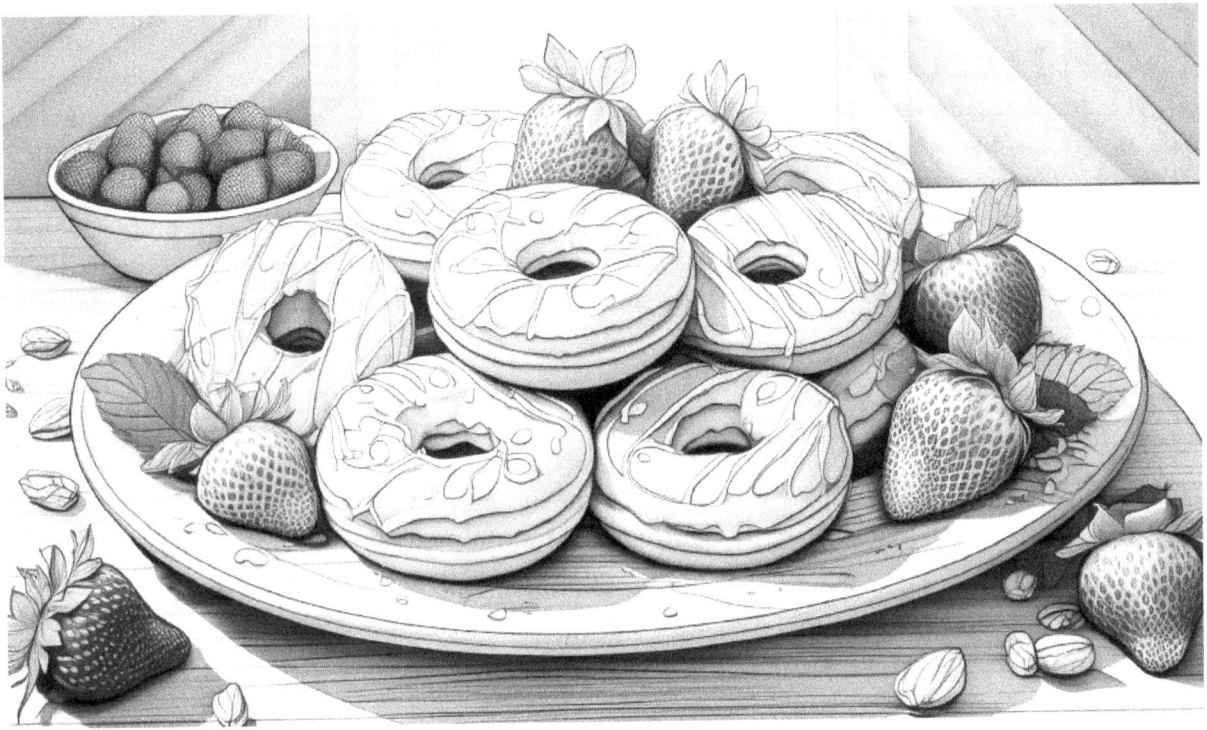

Filling

Nutrition Facts

Serving size: As much as you want in moderation
Servings: 12

Amount per serving
Calories 577

	% Daily Value*
Total Fat 6.9g	9%
Saturated Fat 0.4g	2%
Cholesterol 0mg	0%
Sodium 18mg	1%
Total Carbohydrate 137.3g	50%
Dietary Fiber 15.6g	56%
Total Sugars 114.2g	
Protein 7.1g	
Vitamin D 0mcg	0%
Calcium 83mg	6%
Iron 3mg	14%
Potassium 1266mg	27%

*The % Daily Value (DV) tells you how much a nutrient in a food serving contributes to a daily diet. 2,000 calorie a day is used for general nutrition advice.

Recipe analyzed by **well**

Crust

Nutrition Facts

Serving size: As much as you want in moderation
Servings: 12

Amount per serving
Calories 333

	% Daily Value*
Total Fat 5.3g	7%
Saturated Fat 0.3g	2%
Cholesterol 0mg	0%
Sodium 14mg	1%
Total Carbohydrate 75.9g	28%
Dietary Fiber 8.6g	31%
Total Sugars 63.4g	
Protein 4.5g	
Vitamin D 0mcg	0%
Calcium 44mg	3%
Iron 1mg	7%
Potassium 700mg	15%

*The % Daily Value (DV) tells you how much a nutrient in a food serving contributes to a daily diet. 2,000 calorie a day is used for general nutrition advice.

Recipe analyzed by **well**

Topping

Nutrition Facts

Serving size: As much as you want in moderation
Servings: 12

Amount per serving
Calories 22

	% Daily Value*
Total Fat 0.2g	0%
Saturated Fat 0g	0%
Cholesterol 0mg	0%
Sodium 2mg	0%
Total Carbohydrate 5.4g	2%
Dietary Fiber 1.1g	4%
Total Sugars 3.7g	
Protein 0.4g	
Vitamin D 0mcg	0%
Calcium 9mg	1%
Iron 0mg	2%
Potassium 78mg	2%

*The % Daily Value (DV) tells you how much a nutrient in a food serving contributes to a daily diet. 2,000 calorie a day is used for general nutrition advice.

Recipe analyzed by **well**

Ch 6: Sips & Sweets : Strawberry Cheesecake

Peanut Butter Dates

Peanut butter dates offer a delightful fusion of rich, creamy peanut butter and the natural sweetness of dates, a fruit with ancient ties to the Americas. Indigenous cultures have long valued dates for their energy-boosting properties and sweet flavor. This treat combines unsalted butter, confectioners sugar, peanut butter, and vanilla extract to create a smooth, luscious filling for the dates. Perfect as a snack or dessert, peanut butter dates celebrate the simple yet indulgent flavors that have been cherished through the centuries. Enjoy this blend of tradition and taste, bringing together the best of natural ingredients in a delicious, satisfying bite.

Ingredients

- 1/2 Cup Unsalted Butter
- 2 Cups Confectioners Sugar
- 1 1/2 Cup Peanut Butter
- 1 Tsp Pure Vanilla Extract
- 1/2 Cup Milk
- 12 - 24 Dates

Step 1

1. In a medium or large bowl mix butter and peanut butter until fully combined forming a smooth paste.
2. Add and mix confectioners sugar until fully incorporated.
3. Next add milk and vanilla extract. Mix well.
4. Last, remove pits from dates (if they aren't pitted), add peanut butter mixture to a piping bag (medium or large freezer bag) and fill dates with the mixture.

Nutrition Facts

Serving size: 1 - 2 Dates
Servings: 12

Amount per serving
Calories 477

% Daily Value*

Total Fat 10.3g	13%
Saturated Fat 2.4g	12%
Cholesterol 0mg	0%
Sodium 101mg	4%
Total Carbohydrate 95.2g	35%
Dietary Fiber 8.7g	31%
Total Sugars 81.9g	
Protein 5.7g	
Vitamin D 0mcg	0%
Calcium 53mg	4%
Iron 2mg	13%
Potassium 750mg	16%

*The % Daily Value (DV) tells you how much a nutrient in a food serving contributes to a daily diet. 2,000 calorie a day is used for general nutrition advice.

Recipe analyzed by verywell

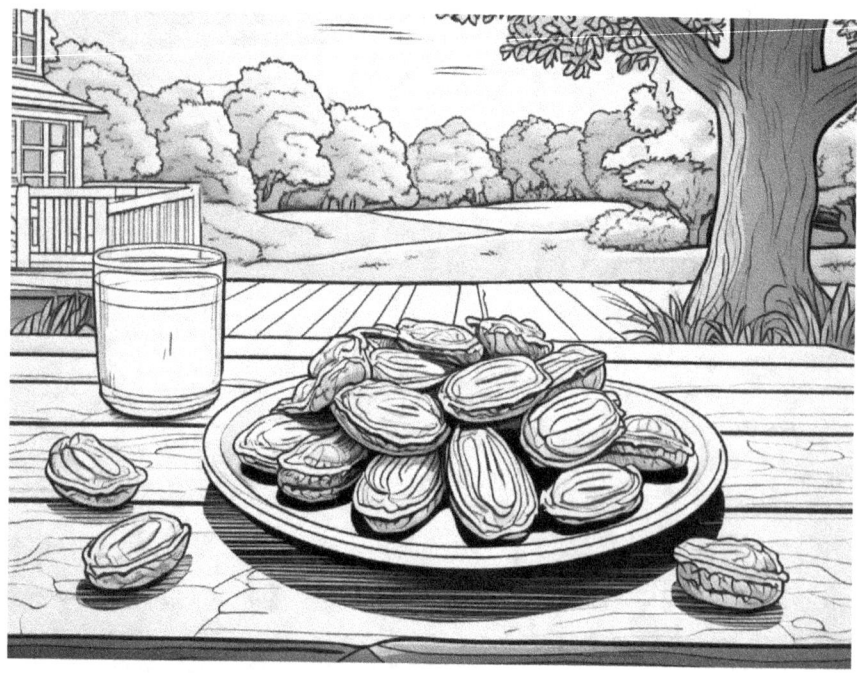

Ch 6: Sips & Sweets : Peanut Butter Dates

Other Titles from Califa Media Publishing

77 Amazing Facts About the Moors with Complete Proof

(C)over Your Head: A Pictographic Chronology of the Moslem Turban

"Watch My Prophesies:" An Examination of Prophesies from the Prophet Noble Drew Ali

Hidden in Plain Sight: The Parable of the Moorish Sardine

Holistic Philosophy 102

Isonomi: The Great Masonic Secret: Master Keys

Moors in America: A Compilation

Moslem Girls Training Guide: Divinely Prepared for the Sisters' Auxiliary of the Moorish Science Temple of America

Mysteries of the Silent Brotherhood the East aka The Red Book

Nationality: The Order of the Day: Divine Message and Warning, All Garveyites, Rastafarians, Black Nationalists & Pan-Africans

Noble Drew Ali Plenipotentiaries

Official Proclamation of Real Moorish American Nationality

The Holy Koran of the Moorish Holy Temple of Science - 1928 Reprint

The Holy Koran of the Moorish Science Temple of America - Hardcover Edition

The Torch: A Guide to Self

Who Stole the Fez, Moors or Shriners

You Are NOT Negro, Black, Coloured, Morisco, Nor an African Slave

www.ingramcontent.com/pod-product-compliance
Lightning Source LLC
Chambersburg PA
CBHW081501070526
44586CB00019B/2455